SEASONS OF CHANGE

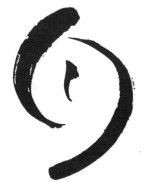

Growing Through Pregnancy & Birth

**Text & Photos
by Suzanne Arms**

Illustrations © 1994 Suzanne Arms, except for the following photographs:
John Arms (pp. 2, 3, 6, 10, bottom of 11, 18, 19, 20, 25, 30, 35, 37, 43, 46, 47, 55, top of
56, 57, top of 68, bottom of 71, top of 72, 98, 104, bottom of 116, 147, left on 168, 174,
top & right on 178)
Molly Arms (pp. 44, 51, 54, 58)
Elliott Kuhner (p. 33)

Kivakí Press
585 East 31st Street
Durango, CO 81301
(303) 385-1767

Library of Congress Catalog Number: 94-076629

Publisher's Cataloging in Publication

Arms, Suzanne.
    Seasons of change : growing through pregnancy and birth /
Suzanne Arms.
    p. cm.
    Preassigned LCCN: 94-076629.
    ISBN 1-88230-858-1

    1. Pregnancy—Psychological aspects. 2. Childbirth—
Psychological aspects. I. Title.

RG560.A792 1994   618.24
                                   QBI94-1338

Book Design: Olive Charles and Suzanne Arms
Cover Design: Olive Charles

Printed in the United States of America
First Edition

Printed on Recycled Paper

First Printing 1994
5 4 3 2   99 98 97 96 95

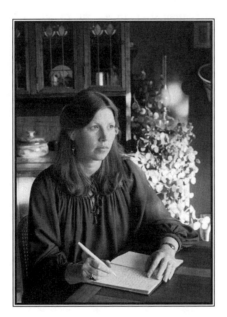

To Molly
with love and gratitude
for all that you continue to teach me
about myself
and the art of mothering

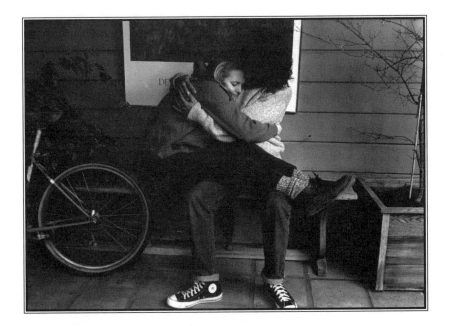

I'm pregnant!

Can I really be?

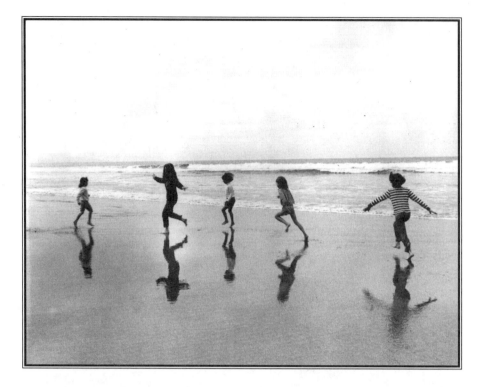

I woke up this morning and it was so beautiful outside. I have been feeling spring in my body for weeks. But now I can see and feel and smell—and hear—spring. It's still cold in the mornings, but the birds are singing. I lay in bed, looking at the patterns the sun was making on my wall. Then it suddenly hit me: I'm pregnant!

I'm in shock.

Is having a baby what I've really wanted—but denied myself—all this time?

I just had to be sure, so I went for
an exam. It's true! The nurse practitioner said my cervix is swollen and
pink and beautiful. I feel like I
brought a brand new body home. A
new me! Only no one knows.

I was pretty sure I must be pregnant last week when I found myself
holding my breasts when I was run-
ning up the stairs. They've been getting much bigger, and sore. My period
was very late, but that's not unusual
for me. Today I bought a new bra, a
whole size bigger.

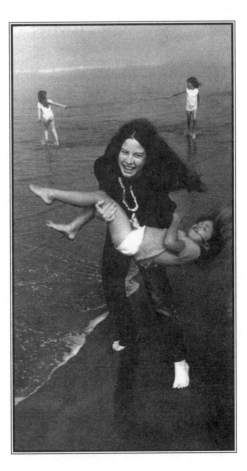

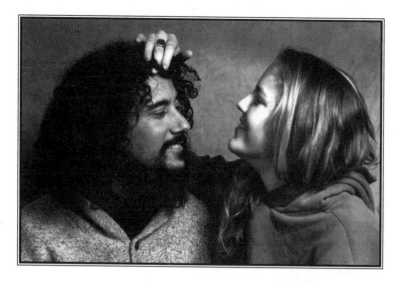

Suddenly, everything's so different. I look at Jay in a whole new way.

Full moon last night. It was so big as it came up. I love the moon. If it weren't so cold out, I would have gone camping just to sleep out underneath it.

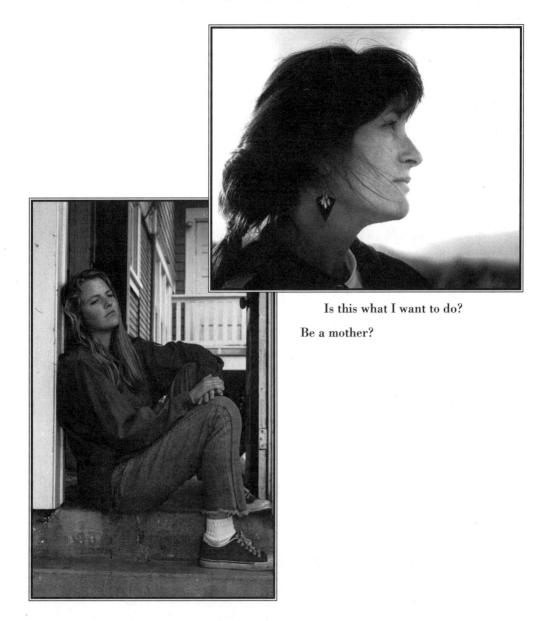

Is this what I want to do?

Be a mother?

I didn't realize that allowing another life to grow in me would take a leap of faith—and daring. I'm always dreaming and planning, trying to imagine and pre-pare for everything. But that just gets you so far. Jay and I have talked about it forever. The pros, the cons. Finally we both agreed: Let's just take the leap! There is no perfect time.

But is this really what I want to do *now*?

Thank God women have a choice today! I can't imagine what it would be like to find out you're pregnant, not want to be, and have no choice about it.

I need to think about this. It's a lot different than I thought it would be, when getting pregnant was just a dream. I'm not used to the idea. How do I *really* feel?

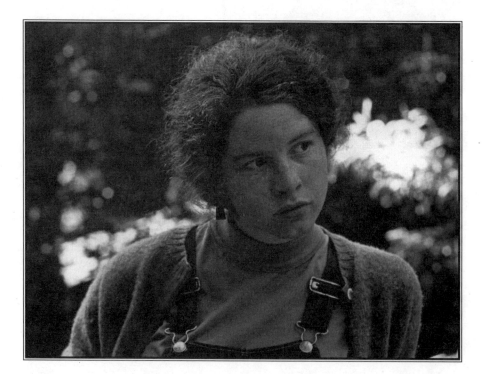

Jay says that he wants to be a dad, and that everything's going to be fine. It's great seeing him so excited. I didn't know how he'd react once it really happened.

I'm glad *he's* sure; but *I'm* not. And today I feel very alone with my feelings. The decision really has to be mine. It's *my* body so I have to feel more responsible.

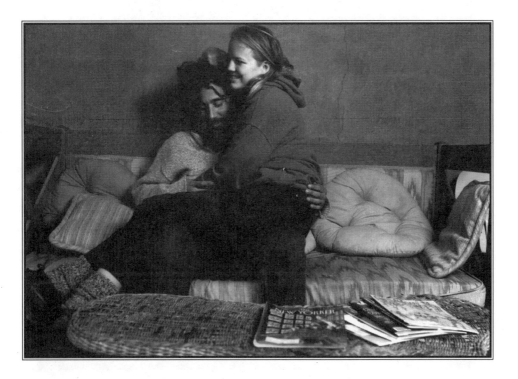

I know lots of women think they'll be with the baby's father forever. Like it's a guarantee once there's a baby. Then they find they're alone, a single mother. I was just listening to some show about welfare and single mothers. People in the audience were talking as if women *want* to be single mothers, and making it sound like it's all the woman's fault if she can't get the father to pay child support and needs public assistance. I've never met a single mother who thought that was the best way to raise a child. I sure don't want to be one. But how can anyone be sure?

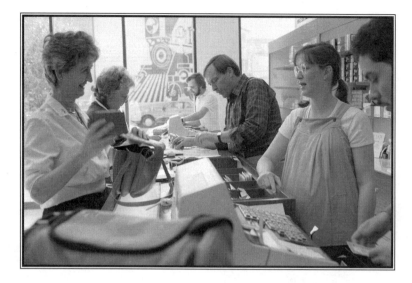

Suddenly, I'm seeing pregnant women everywhere.

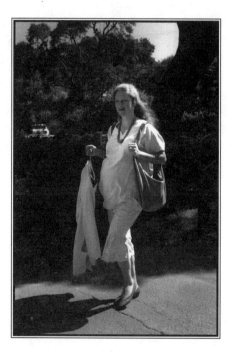

This is what I want. It's the biggest decision I've ever had to make. This baby won't be just an extension of me. It will be a whole other person I'll have to be responsible for. Can I— do I really *want* to—do this? Now?

I know if I do become a parent, I'll give it everything I have. I know it won't be like baby-sitting. It's being responsible for someone 24 hours a day. Having to be there for someone who really needs you, whose future is in your hands.

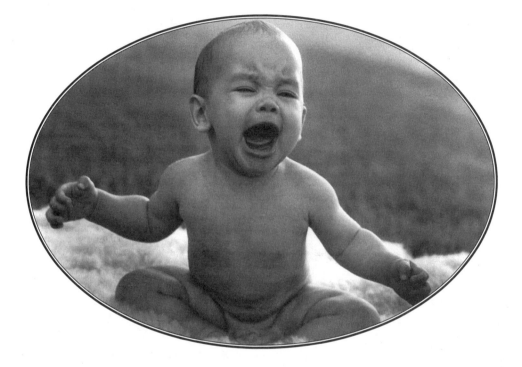

I used to think sometimes it would be wonderful to have a baby, someone to take care of, someone who would love me totally. But how do you take care of a baby all the time, love it all the time, even when it's screaming?

YES! I will! Yes!

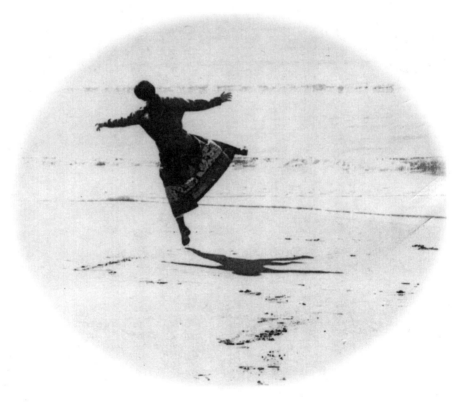

Jay's so glad I finally committed to this pregnancy. I think for a while he wanted it even more than I and would have been really sad if we didn't have this baby. If he thinks *he's* glad, he should be in *my* body!

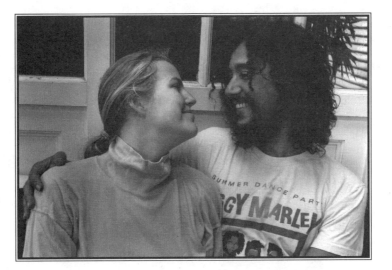

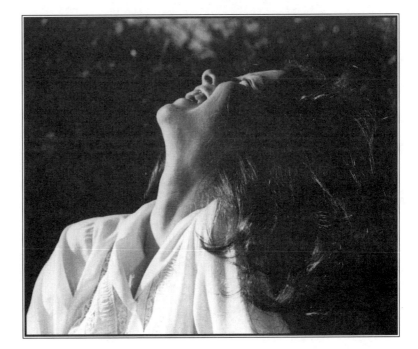

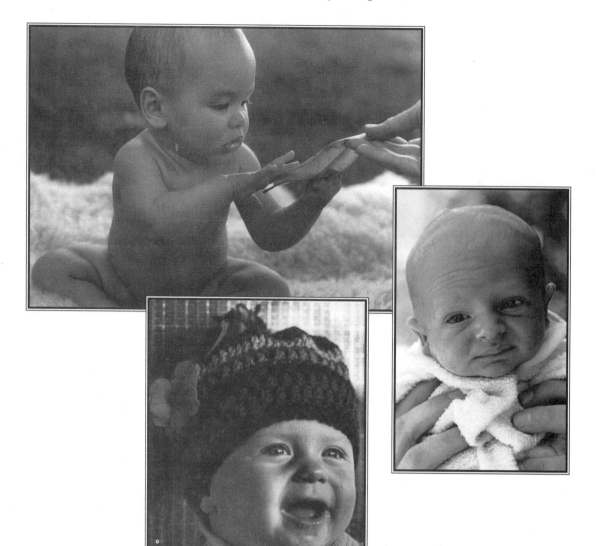

I've been around other people's children. There have been times when I couldn't stand someone's kid, didn't even want to be around *any*. But there have always been a few whom I felt that special connection with. It didn't have anything to do with whether they were related to me, or how long I'd known them. Some kids—and some babies—have just reached in and grabbed my heart.

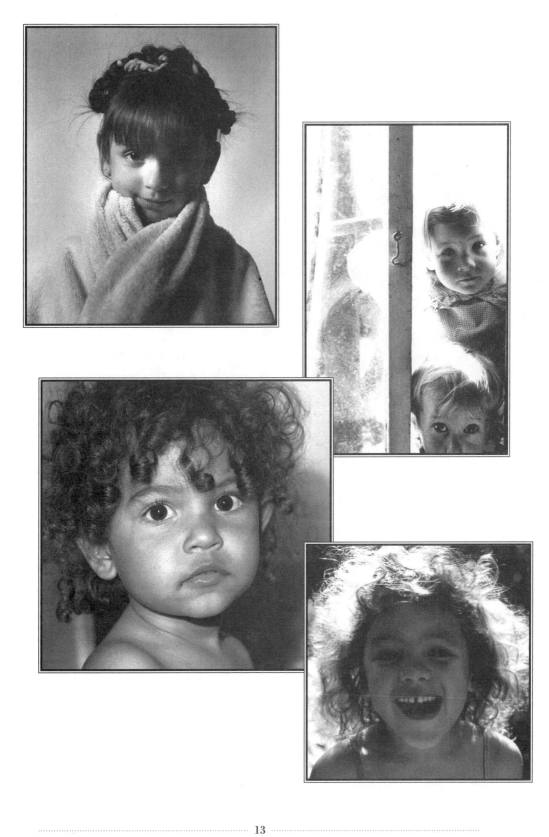

Sometimes, when I'm half-asleep or just waking up, I feel like a baby's spirit is hovering around me. I've never felt anything like this. No one I know has ever talked about it. Is it this baby's spirit? If so, I want it to know that I'm so glad it's chosen to come to me. I promise I'll be the best mother I can.

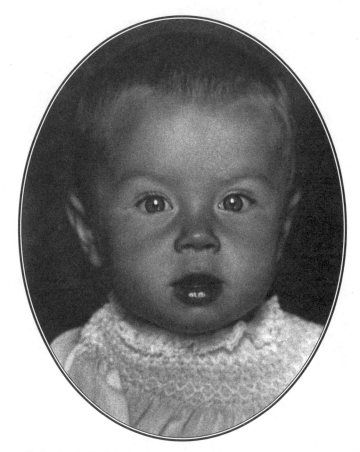

What will this baby be like? When we look at each other the first time, will we already know each other?

Just before sunset I saw a flock of geese flying north in a perfectly straight line. Sometimes I wish I could fly.

I wonder if every woman who's pregnant with her first baby feels like I do, that I'm the very first woman ever to feel what I am feeling?

I want to know what pregnancy is like for women in other parts of the world—not the modern world, but in tribes and villages. I don't feel like I belong where I am right now. So much pavement. Having to leave my home five days a week to go to work, where nobody talks about the kinds of things I want to talk about now, all the things I'm thinking and feeling.

I'm in a magic circle. No one can touch this life inside of me. We're protected.

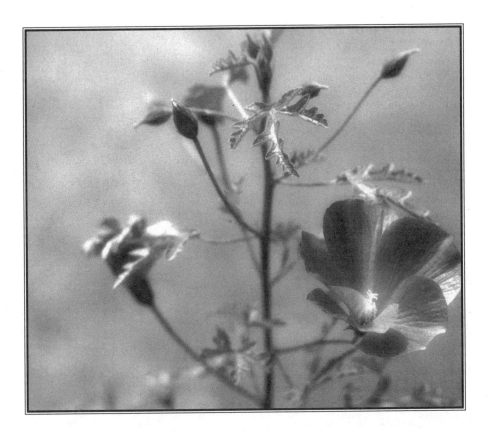

The weather is moody this week and the sky is gray. My moods are shifting fast. I guess it's hormones. I've never felt so vulnerable. That bubble of protection I was feeling so strongly just a few days ago, where did it go?

Can I really count on Jay to be there? For me? And for our baby? Or will he leave some day when things are tough?

Will he be a good father? What am I talking about? Will *I* be able to do it? Will *I* be a good enough mother?

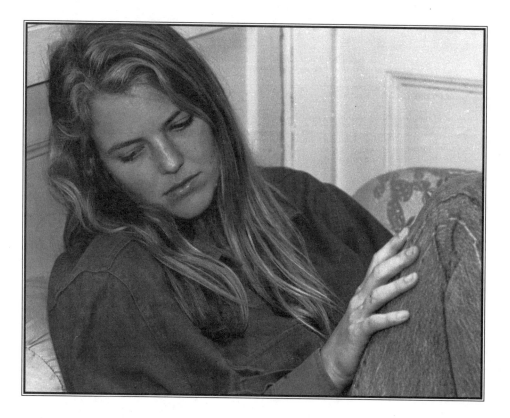

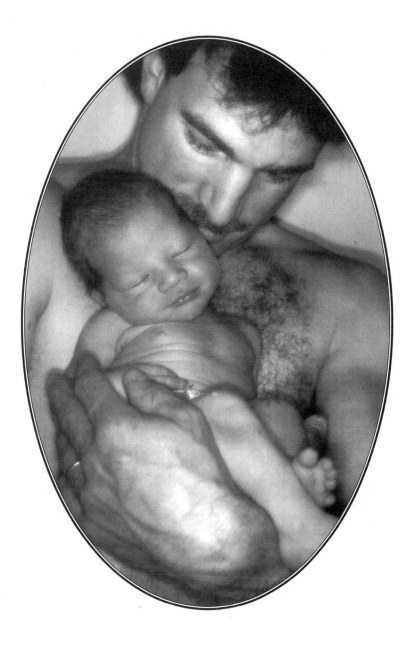

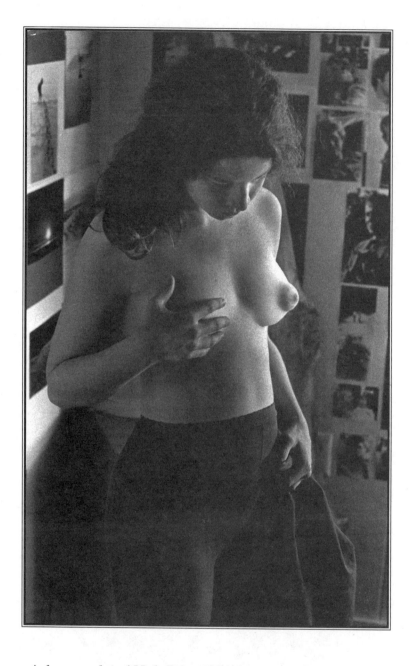

At last, a real sign! My belly's still flat but my nipples are swollen and getting darker. What an amazing thing to happen to my body.

I'm so happy today. I've been
dancing around our apartment. Just
being alive makes me want to shout,
Thank you!

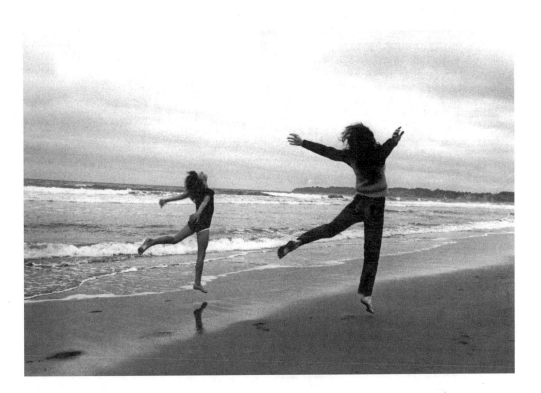

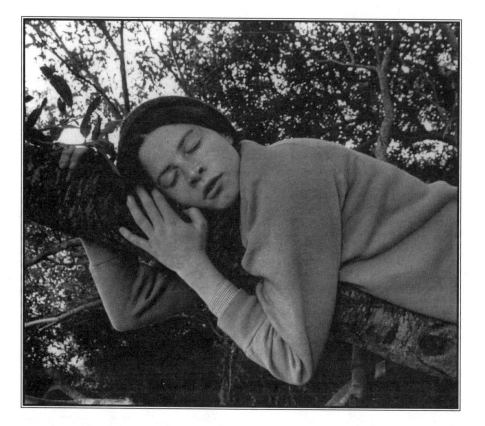

There are certain places that have always made me feel at peace. That's where I go when I feel disconnected and need to feel whole. That's where I want to be right now, not on the third floor of some concrete building, wearing "go-to-work" clothes!

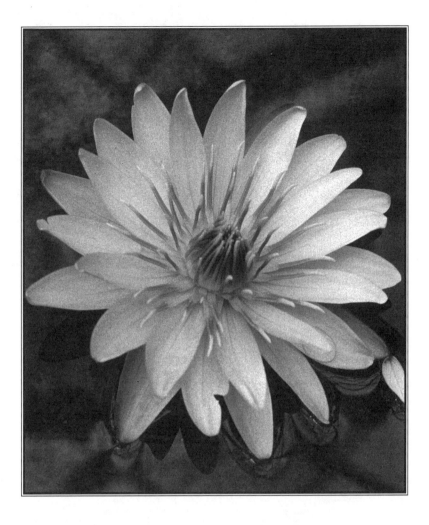

I drove to the conservatorium today and spent two hours wandering through the different rooms—some hot and dry climates, some moist and warm. I've always loved roses, especially the old-fashioned ones that smell so strong. I'd like to grow roses. I loved the orchids I saw, even though they have no smell. In the orchid room there was a feeling of warm mist on my skin, like someone's gentle touch. But my favorite was the room with the pond with the lily pads. The blossoms are so white against the green leaves in the dark water. I sat and gazed into the water for a long time, and felt myself come back together again.

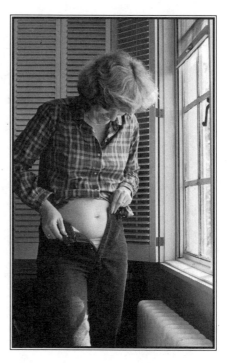

I'm on a path and there's no turning back. It's so different from anything else I've known. I wonder if every pregnant woman feels this way.

Today I couldn't get my old jeans to button at all. My belly doesn't look very different yet. But there's a hard round spot below my navel. Is that my uterus?

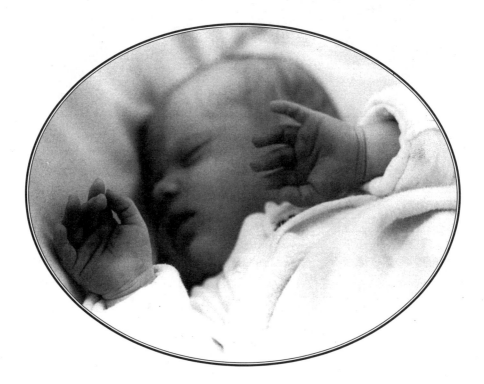

It's weird. Something—something that will be *someone*—growing inside me. Already with tiny hands and feet. Inside me.

Now I have to be stable. There's another *person* to think about. Another person who will be with me every day. What a responsibility!

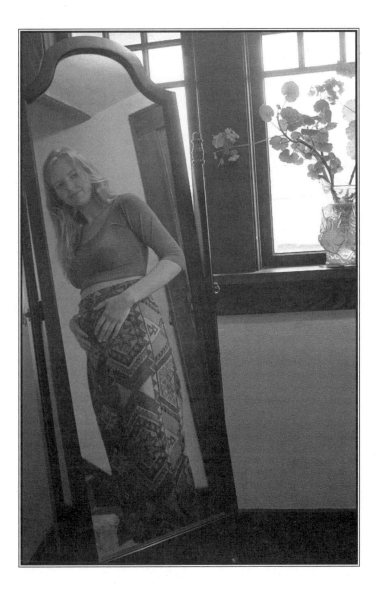

My head is full of thoughts. I am filled with questions. But I don't know who to ask or what I'd even say. It's not something I want to share with Jay. Not today. I think I'll go buy a blank book and start a diary.

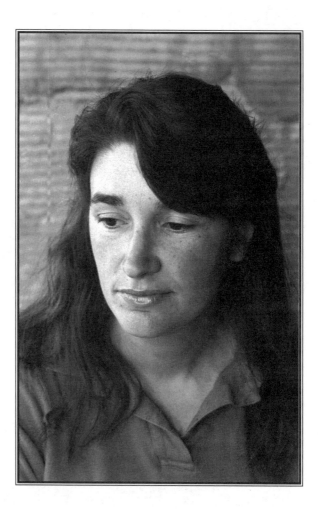

It's strange, Jay and I are so close. Yet, sometimes, when I am lying in bed with him, I feel so far apart.

When will I feel the baby moving inside me? Kim says it won't be for at least three months, maybe four. That's too long to wait!

If I could just have some more signs—I'd even be glad to have morning sickness. Then I could believe it's real.

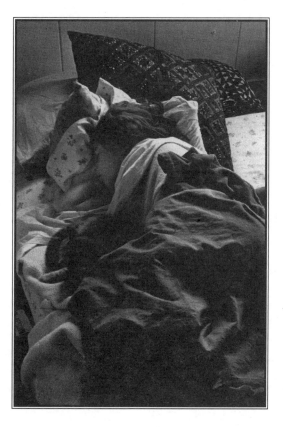

Nausea! For almost a week. There's nothing worse. Why do they call it "morning sickness"? I feel it all day long. As a kid I always hated to throw up. I sure wish I could throw up now.

I must be pregnant. I feel so sick.

There were several big-bellied women in the waiting room at my first prenatal visit. They looked at me like I was in the wrong place. I want to look like them! I can't wait to have to buy something new because none of my clothes will fit. Only I wish I didn't feel so sick.

Peppermint tea. Mint-flavored chewing gum. Ice cold fizzy mineral water. Ginger ale. Chamomile tea. Plain saltine crackers. I try everything anyone suggests. They all help a bit. People are right, it is good to keep something in my stomach, especially something salty. But every morning when I wake up, the nausea is right there. And it hardly ever goes away completely. I sure don't feel sexy.

It feels like I'm constantly about to throw up, like there's something in my throat and I'm about to gag. But I can't. Some days I can throw up. Yesterday my stomach muscles ached from doing it too much, and there was nothing in my stomach but bitter stuff. I'm so glad I didn't start out real thin. I've *lost* weight. I'd give anything to be able to eat and put on some. For the baby.

I've always loved to eat. Now I hate the thought of food.

I just talked to a woman at work who has two kids. I remember her saying she had morning sickness with her second for three months. She said it usually goes away on its own by the end of the first three months. But she found vitamin B6 helped a lot. She read that pregnant women in modern countries tend to be low on that vitamin. I'll get some. I'll do anything that works!

I called Michelle. She had a midwife for her pregnancy in Michigan. I remember her being nauseous for a long time. She said her midwife told her about ginger root. It worked for her. She said I can get it powdered in bulk at a health food store and buy empty glycerin capsules, fill them, and take as much as I like because it doesn't have any side effects.

I have to be so careful now. I have another life to think about. I think I'll go get some fresh ginger and put slices in boiling water, make a tea. Maybe with honey and lemon. That sounds good. Nothing else has worked today.

Last night I couldn't sleep because I was going over and over in my mind everything I did—and ate and drank—for the past couple of months, before I knew. I couldn't stand it if I knew that something I've done might hurt this baby.

I just want to sleep all day. At least I don't feel the nausea when I'm asleep. I can't stand the smell of most foods—even my favorites—or watching anyone eat.

I've lost all track of time. Last night, when I couldn't go right to sleep, and Jay was lying there out like a light, I sat out on the steps and watched the stars. Only the street lights were on, so I could see more stars. The feeling of the cool air on my skin and in my nose made the nausea less, too. Looking at the sky reminded me how lucky I am to be alive. Thank you, God, for all my blessings.

I just read that nausea in early pregnancy usually goes with a healthy fetus and can be a sign that the fertilized egg has implanted itself well into the lining of the uterus. That's great! But it seems counter-productive to me. I lost a pound last week. How's this baby ever going to get nourished, if I'm too sick to eat? Do women in tribal cultures get so nauseous they can't eat? Or is this just another part of modern life?

I don't want to see anybody. I don't want to talk to anybody. I don't want to do anything. I'm so tired all the time. I told Jay, if this nausea is going to last the whole pregnancy, I can't do it! I can't imagine being a mother, taking care of a baby 24 hours a day. How do people take care of a baby when they are really sick? I just want to crawl in a cave somewhere or be babied myself.

Thank God it's Saturday. There's nothing I have to do. How do women do it who can't take time off of work when they're this nauseous! I have so much respect for mothers.

The nausea seems milder the last few days. Maybe it's going away. I don't dare get excited, just in case. Last week was my twelve week visit. Today I felt good enough to take a walk right after I got up. And then I actually ate breakfast with Jay. Boy, was he surprised! This pregnancy has sure been hard on us these past few weeks. It's changing our relationship.

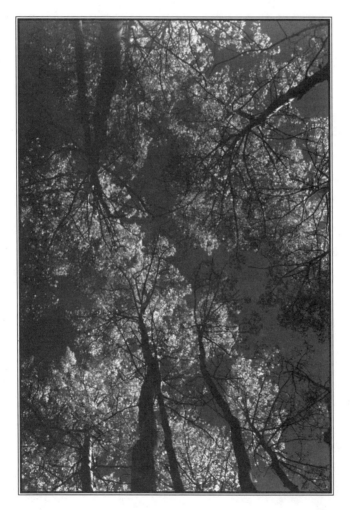

At last! No morning sickness for five whole days! I feel alive again!

I still can't even think about eat-ing the foods that made me vomit a few weeks ago. They were some of my favorite foods. The memory is too vivid. I can still feel it.

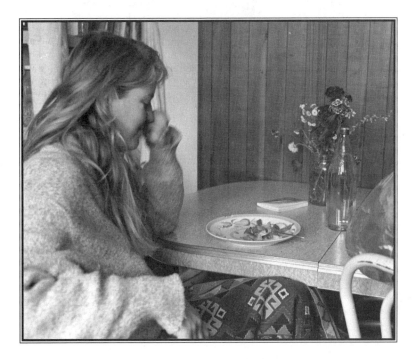

Now that I'm not sick, I'm so excited. I can't stop thinking about the mira-cle of it all. I don't want to go to work today and fill my mind with other things. This baby! Inside me! I want to stop people on the street and tell them.

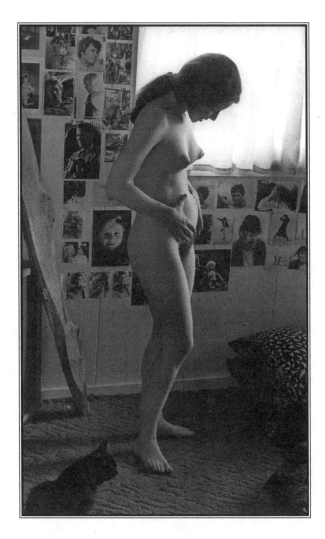

Finally, I'm putting on some weight for this baby!

I just read that a pregnant woman's body has to grow hundreds of miles of new capillaries to handle all the extra blood her body must make to grow and carry a healthy baby. Amazing! I'm eating every chance I can get. I'm *so* hungry. I asked my doctor how much I should let myself gain. She says it's normal for a woman to gain twenty-five or thirty pounds by the end of pregnancy, but that she doesn't want me to gain much more than that.

Today I went and bought my first maternity outfit! One day I'll fill it. I can't imagine what that will be like.

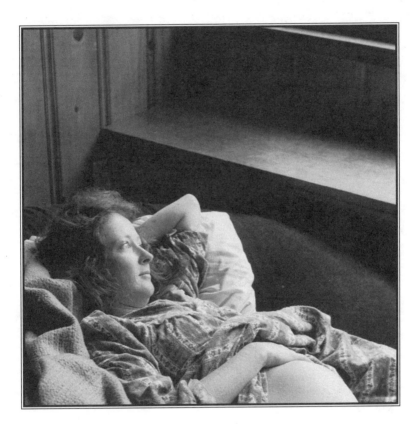

It's the middle of the night. Jay is asleep. I can't fall asleep. There is no moon, the sky is pitch black and I can't see the stars.

I feel so lonely. It rained today. Usually I love the smell of everything wet from the rain. But right now, I feel far away from everything warm and safe. I'm floating in blackness.

Will holding this baby in my arms keep me from ever being lonely again?

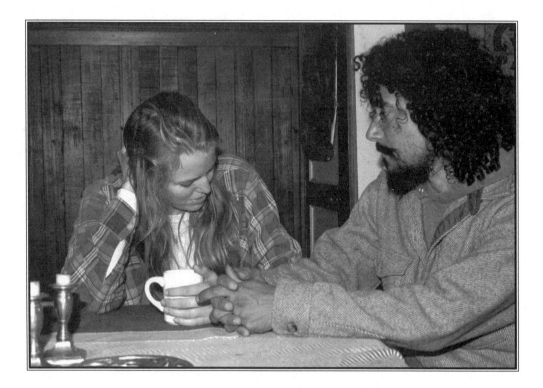

Jay and I have been arguing a lot lately. I hate it. Mostly it's about money. Also, we just found out we have to move. This place isn't light enough anyway. I want a place full of light for this baby. But where will we get the money?

It just hit me. I've thought so much about being a mother, but not at all about the birth. To have a baby I have to go through labor. I'm a real wimp about pain. Can I get through without taking drugs? I want to. I don't want to miss any part of it. Mom and I've talked about that. She agrees. She had a lot of drugs when she had me. She didn't want them, but they pushed and she gave in. And she was sorry. She said that my face showed the effects of the drugs when I was born. My eyes weren't clear and bright. And I was very sleepy nursing for the first week. I know natural childbirth is best for the baby. But I'm scared.

At last! I've begun to feel the baby moving. At least, I'm pretty sure it's the baby. It feels more like a little fluttering—or a small fish swimming around beneath my belly button. It's weird. I like it.

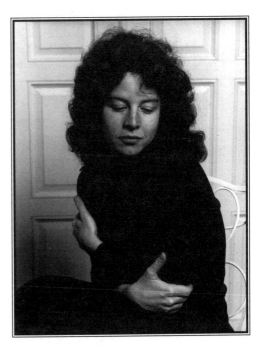

What is this birth going to be like? How can I prepare for something so different from anything I've ever known? I guess *every* experience is really just like this—totally new, and something you can't really prepare for. But birth seems so different. I can't relate it to anything.

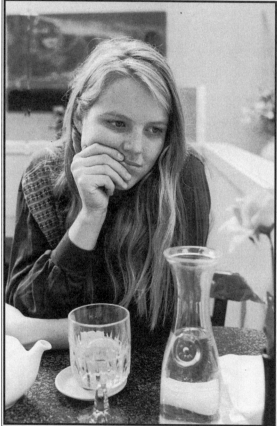

At the library most of the books on birth were out, but I found an old copy of a book Mom mentioned, called *Childbirth Without Fear*. It was written in the 1940s by a British doctor named Grantly Dick-Read. I'm sure things have changed a lot since then, but mom said it really inspired her, and a lot of other women too. I looked at the stamped dates showing how often it's been taken out, and nobody has taken it out for almost a year.

I've read nearly half of my book already. It's about natural childbirth and how women all over the world have been able to have healthy babies without any help whatsoever—and no drugs— and still come through it feeling good about their birth. When he was a doctor in England and saw women having babies in their own homes, Read met a lot of working class women who refused any drugs because they knew they could do it on their own. He also went to rural Africa and got to see women there having babies. He noticed that they also did really well in labor, even with the pain.

That book really made me think. It's given me some confidence, too.

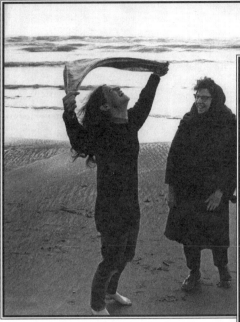

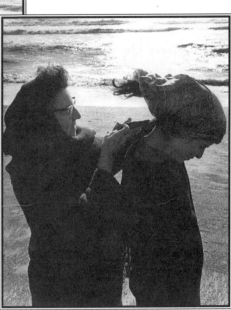

My mom and I had another long talk today. Right now I wish we lived next door to each other. That's a change! I told her I'm pretty sure I want to have natural childbirth. She said she'll do anything she can to help, that she really thinks it's important. Not only for the woman to discover how capable and powerful she is, but also because the baby isn't meant to have any drugs in its body when it's born. It needs all of its senses fully functioning to experience the world. Most drugs have side effects for the baby, including breathing problems. The baby gets whatever the mother takes in, through the umbilical cord. That did it for me. Somehow, I'll manage to do it without drugs.

Mom said when she told her mother that's what she wanted she said, "You're crazy!" What's crazy about wanting to feel everything about the miracle of a baby coming out of your body and wanting to give your baby the best start?

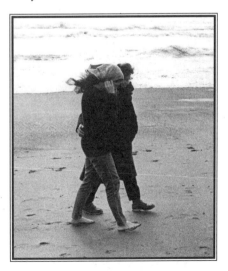

I had another talk with mom over the weekend. She told me some about her birth—*my* birth—and the anger and sadness she felt after a few months, when she began thinking about all the things they did to her in labor and how she didn't fight. Only years later did she start thinking about what *my* experience must have been like, and then she felt very bad that she didn't protect me from all the drugs and other things. It was because contraction hurt so much, and she was frightened. Plus, she just wanted to please everyone. She told me that's how she made it through childhood, by pleasing everyone, and when labor began she fell right back into that old pattern. She said she didn't feel like she really had any choices, because the nurses and doctors had a certain idea in mind about what they wanted to do and they pushed it.

She doesn't think most women, even today, really make conscious choices about their births. They have so much fear about the pain and don't want to experience what's happening, so they opt for drugs or anesthesia, even cesarean, just to get through it the "easiest" way. I'm glad I don't feel that way. I'm just scared about what it'll be like.

I feel bad for Mom about her birth with me. And I feel kind of sad now that I think about what it was like for me, as a baby. I wish it had been different. I wish a lot of things had been different about my childhood. I know it was really hard in the years when my mother was a single mom, getting no child support and feeling overwhelmed and having a lot of depressions. I'm so glad she breastfed me for a long time. She said she was certain it made up for a lot of what went wrong in the birth. I want this baby to have an easier start in life.

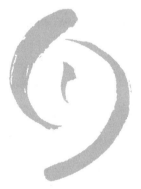

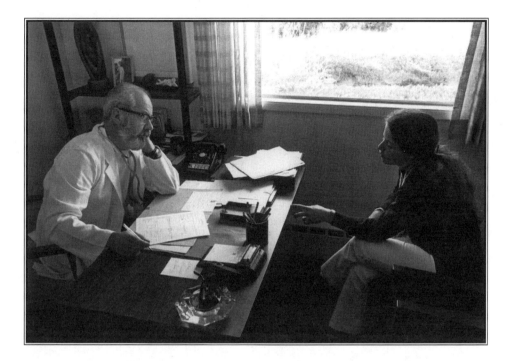

My mom asked me if I was still wanting to have a natural birth. When I told her I am, she said it's real important that I have good support in labor from people around. She didn't have that. My dad was there and stayed the whole time, but he agreed with the nurses that she should take drugs, and told her she didn't have to be a martyr. She asked if my doctor really supported natural childbirth, because that would make a lot of difference. I don't know what my doctor really thinks. I've only seen her a couple times and she's very nice.

I've been thinking about the things my mother said all week, so I called her again. Suddenly I just want to know *everything*! I wish I'd had a better birth, but at least I know she really wanted me and had a pretty happy pregnancy. She said, in pregnancy, whenever she got into an argument with my dad or felt depressed, she worried about what it might be doing to me. That's the way I feel.

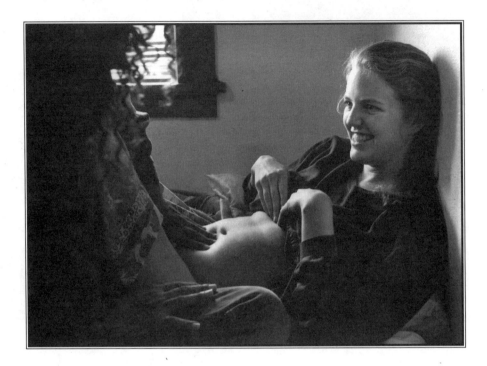

I'm just starting a book I bought about the intelligence and consciousness of babies—in the womb as well as at birth. It's fascinating. Apparently, it's not whether the mother has some bad times or is even depressed sometimes in pregnancy. It's *overall* that matters. That's what the baby feels. Especially the relationship between the mother and father, or whoever else the mother is living with. That makes sense. I don't know why they don't teach this in schools. Why doesn't anyone talk about it?

Everyone seems to believe that it's the age from two to five that's so important, as if what happens before a baby can talk doesn't really matter, or is forgotten. According to the research in *this* book, babies *know* what is going on, even at conception. And we don't forget our birth. The memories are there, inside us, still affecting us. Wow!

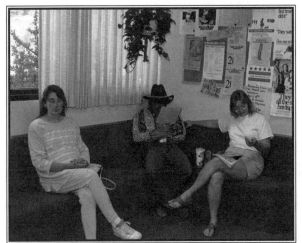

Mom says women have been giving their bodies over to doctors in this country—especially when it comes to birth—for a long time. I think I know why. It's scary going into something unknown, where you know there's going to be pain and some real risk. And almost everyone talks about how awful it is and how risky it is. I find myself wanting my doctor to know everything and be the expert, just to be able to lean on someone else. I just don't feel sure of myself.

Mom said her mother had taught her to always do whatever your doctor thinks is best because doctors are trained to know. We both laughed about that. But it's not really funny. I'd like to find out about great Grandma Brady's births. Mom's going to ask Grandma and see what she remembers. I feel like a detective.

I'm starting to think about birth classes. I can't believe how fast this pregnancy is going! I asked mom if she went to classes. She did, because she wanted to learn how to have a natural birth. There weren't many classes to choose from in 1970, and her Lamaze teacher spent most of the class having everyone practice special kinds of breathing, which one to do for each part of labor. She said her teacher made birth into some kind of athletic event you had to train for, and breathe in a certain way, or you wouldn't get it right. She said there was a lot about medication, too; all the different kinds of drugs and anesthesia and all the things that can go wrong in birth. But there was nothing about the bad effects of drugs on the labor or on the baby. She dropped out of the class after a few weeks.

Where she lived, in Northern California, there were some home births going on. It was 1970, and some women were becoming lay midwives to help other women have home births. She said she really wanted to go to one, or at least see a natural birth in a hospital. One woman planning to have a natural birth invited her to go with her to the hospital, but the nurses refused to let her be there. Another woman invited her to her home birth, but some guy who was a roommate was disgusted by the idea and insisted she go to the hospital. So Mom never did get to see any birth, except a film of a hospital birth with the woman all covered in drapes and lying on her back with her legs up in the air strapped down in stirrups and her hands in handcuffs.

Mom said she purposely chose a group of doctors—all men, because that's how it was then—who had a reputation for supporting natural childbirth. The hospital they used was thirty miles from where she and Dad lived. Dad was allowed to stay with her in labor. That was apparently a big deal in those days; no one but the father could be there with you. Hospital policy. Anyway, she ended up going to the hospital too early, at only 1 centimeter dilated, because her water had broken and that's what the doctor wanted. Also, she was scared to stay at home with contractions.

She wishes she had stayed home, because once she was in the hospital they started doing things to her. She was put into a bed—it was in the basement of the hospital, so there weren't any windows—and the nurse immedi-

ately gave her a shot. Didn't even ask her permission. Just said, "You're nervous!" like that was dumb, and stuck it in. After that it was one thing after another: sedatives, pain medication, artificial hormones to make contractions stronger. She said some of the stuff they gave her isn't even used any more because it was found to cause such serious problems for a lot of babies. She had all she could do to cope with the contractions, lying in bed. Nobody told her contractions hurt more when you lie down and aren't as good at dilating the cervix. But that's what everyone did in those days, she said, the nurses wanted you in bed.

Anyway, she got to 5 centimeters and the nurse said the doctor wanted her to have some kind of spinal anesthesia. She didn't want it, but she took it. It was novocaine into the nerves all around the spinal cord. For some reason the anesthetic didn't work right and ended up stopping labor. So they had to give her a lot more hormones to get it going. She ended up pushing for two hours, but I was stuck—something about the spinal caused it—and I never came down with the pushing. The third doctor in the group—the one she liked the best—did the birth and ended up having to use forceps and pull me out. She said he did it very slowly because he didn't want to hurt me. And I didn't have any marks from the forceps. But she got an awful spinal headache that hurt for two weeks every time she sat or stood up.

She said breast feeding me was wonderful—the best part of it all—because she really knew she was doing something important for me, and it felt good too. She said she's always felt that how I was born made a difference and that it wasn't a good way to begin life. I agree. But she did her best.

I have so many questions about birth. Jay is not much help. But neither are most of the women I know at work who've had babies. They all took drugs and are glad they did. But all my detective work got Jay interested in his family. It turns out his mother's births were pretty easy and two of them were without any drugs, which apparently was real unusual in the late 1960s.

☾

My mom just wrote me a long letter about what she knows about grandma's birth with her. All my questions have gotten her interested in knowing more! Poor grandma! Her mom was all alone in labor. Grandpa was away in the war and no one was allowed with her. There was a shortage of nurses and doctors. Grandma told her the pain seemed unbearable, that she'd make a fist so hard her nails would cut into her palms, just to take her mind off the contractions. She doesn't remember everything and must have had drugs. But she was awake for pushing.

After her first birth grandma was very angry at her mother for not having told her anything about labor ahead of time, but she found out that no one had told Great Grandma Brady anything either. Women kept a lot of secrets from their daughters in those days.

The first experience Grandma had with birth was at the end of her pregnancy with my uncle, when one of her college friends had a baby and she went to see her in the hospital. She couldn't believe how bad her friend looked. Her voice was gone from screaming—that's what she whispered to Grandma, that it was the worst thing that ever happened to her. Grandma didn't get to see the baby because it was in the nursery, with all the other babies. She said she always wondered why women seem to like to tell horror stories about birth.

Anyway, Grandma's doctor was late getting to the hospital and the nurses weren't supposed to let a baby be born before the doctor came. So one of them held Grandma's legs together and the other kept pushing the baby's head back to keep it from coming out. Grandma said all she wanted to do was push the baby out and it hurt really bad not to be able to.

Mom ended up okay but had to be in the nursery for a week because there was an epidemic of infant diarrhea going around and the doctors thought keeping the mothers and babies separated was the best thing. She said she was lucky because she was the first girl baby to have been born in that hospital in many days, so she got lots of attention from the nurses. Wow!

I've been trying to imagine what it must have been like for Mom, as a baby being born, to be trying and trying to come out of her mother's body and be pushed back. I'd have felt desperate. She says she thinks that's a lot of the reason why she has always gone at life with her head, as if she had to push her way through everything. I don't think it's funny. It makes me angry.

I've decided to ask all the women I know what the births have been like in their families. I just can't believe the human race would have continued if it was meant to be this hard and this bad.

One of the women I just met at work said she isn't afraid of birth. Her mother told her it was the hardest work she'd ever done but that it was the most *wonderful* experience of her life. Her mother grew up on a dairy farm. Apparently all the births in her mom's family were normal. There were fourteen kids, they were all born naturally, and all fourteen lived! What a great story!

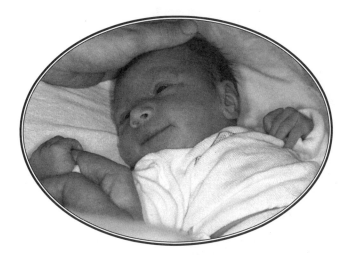

Where are you, Baby? Can you hear my thoughts? I long to hold you and to show you the world.

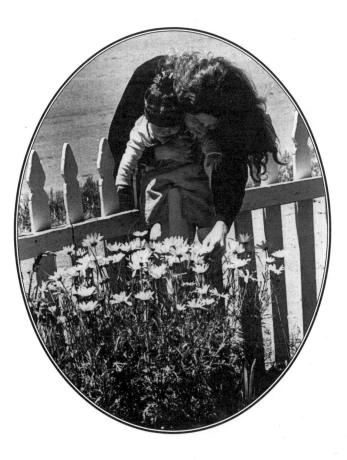

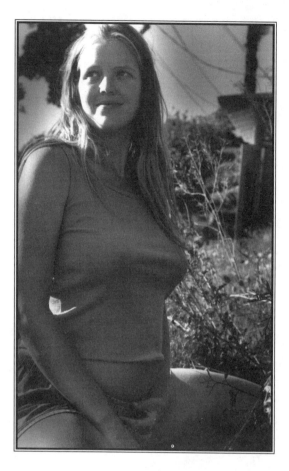

We've been looking at apartments all weekend. Everything's so expensive. We didn't find anything. I hate looking, finding places that are dingy and overpriced or nice but something we can't afford. But I know it's better to move now than have to move right after you have a baby, or when it's just about to come. I need to know where we will be living, so I can settle in.

As long as I have enough food and clothes and a warm place to live, we'll be fine.

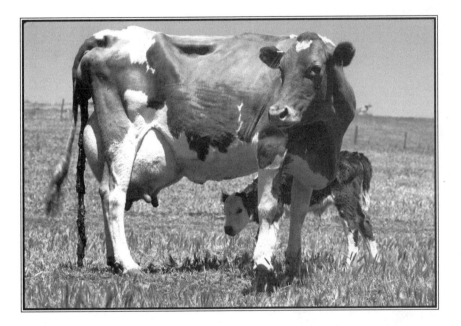

The weather is beautiful these days. I made a picnic, with a checkered table cloth and everything, and we drove out into the country on one of my favorite roads. You'll never guess what we saw! A cow, standing in a pasture right alongside the road, had just had a baby and the afterbirth was still hanging out of her. The calf was just trying to stand up. It was all wet and wobbly and adorable. And the afterbirth was messy-looking, with strings of it hanging out of the mother. That's the first almost-birth I've ever seen.

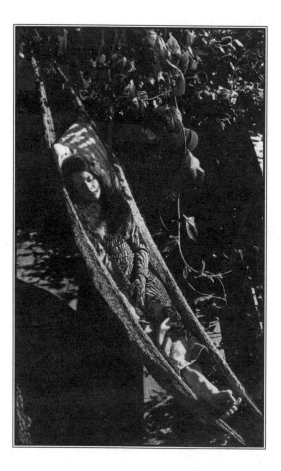

We didn't have much money a lot of time I was growing up, and mom was irritable and depressed a lot. But I always felt she loved me, and I remember her hugging me a lot and apologizing when she blew up. Mom's mom, Grandma Davis, was the super-woman type. She remembers Grandma doing *everything*: working full time, keeping the house clean, shopping, doing all the cooking, helping each of the kids with homework every night, and then staying up till midnight to mark papers, because she was a school teacher.

Mom said her mother never showed her feelings—never got angry, and never sad—and never *ever* relaxed. She said her best memories of Grandma were when she was scared to go to sleep at night and her mom would let her put her head in her lap and would fuss with her head and play with her hair. She said she loved those times, but they weren't often. Grandma was just too busy. I don't want to be like that with this baby. Jay says his mom was really there for him, and only worked part time until he was in first grade. But his dad wasn't. He was always working.

I want to be a kid, not a parent. I want to be taken care of. Not to have to do things for someone else all the time.

My face is really puffed up. I've been crying. I sure cry easily these days. Jay can't even say one word the wrong way without my bursting into tears. I'm so emotional.

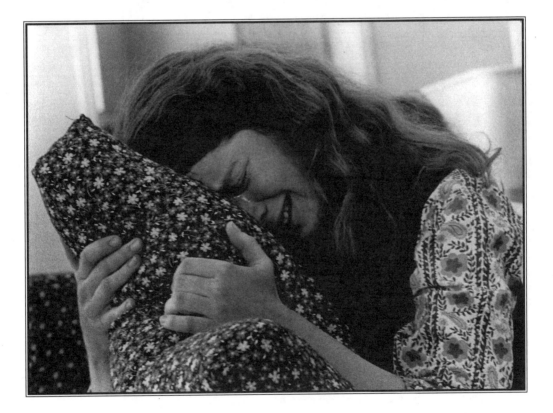

It's my hormones, Mom says. Aren't hormones great?

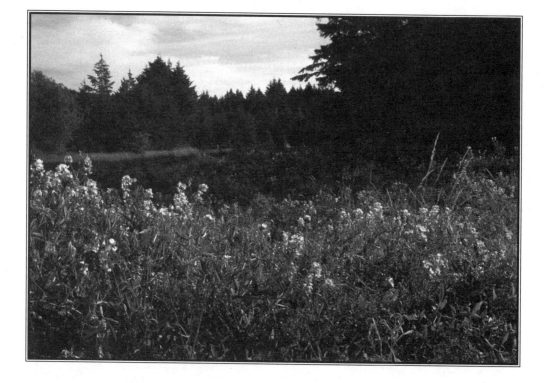

I went for a drive on Saturday. Jay was out at a game with his friends. I found the most beautiful field—it must have been an old orchard, because there were lots of trees in rows. The trees were full of white blossoms and the ground was covered in yellow, I think it's wild mustard. I sat with my back up against a tree, and daydreamed. All my tension drained into the earth—why don't I do this more often?

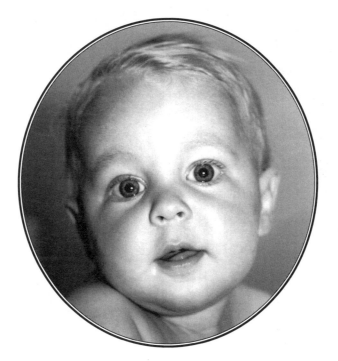

I want this baby to be perfect. Am I doing things right? Sometimes I just want someone to tell me what I have to do and promise that everything will then be all right. Now I know why women have listened to doctors all these years! I'm so unsure of *myself*.

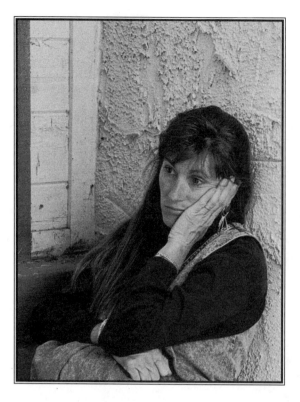

I hate it when there's any strain between Jay and me. Sometimes it's over money, sometimes it's about sex. There are times when I just don't want to and Jay really does, and I feel pressured. And other times when he doesn't, but I do. Mostly my mind's on other things.

Now there's a whole other person to think about. I want to be calm, for the sake of this little person inside. I don't want this baby to be afraid and upset.

Boy, this is a big responsibility. Sometimes I just want to forget about the baby and do whatever I want, and go partying. But then I imagine myself as the baby. What do you need me to do, Baby?

I'm making a lifetime commitment to this baby. I'd like to think Jay and I will be together forever. That's my ideal. Is it too much to expect?

Some of my friends who have kids are married. Some aren't. I've noticed that it doesn't really seem to make much difference whether you're married or not, when it comes to having bad arguments or being totally committed to working things out. There are no guarantees.

Jay and I had a good long talk last night about the future. He's been worried about our arguments, too. We agreed that if we can't find a way through our differences, we'll see a counselor. Jay doesn't like the idea, but he agreed. It's not something his parents ever did. But there's a lot they don't talk about.

We made a promise that, no matter what, if we couldn't make it as a couple, we'd find a way to get along, and share parenting, for the sake of this child. We might even live in the same neighborhood. It's hard to talk about things like this—I don't like thinking about it, but we both agree on how important it is to think of what our child needs.

We're still arguing about little things. I don't know what's going on. I don't even know whose fault it is. My emotions are like a roller coaster and I'm over-sensitive. Jay says he never knows who he's going to meet when I walk in the door. Neither do I!

I'm the whole world for this baby right now. Sometimes it's too much responsibility.

Jay and I went to garage sales this morning. We found a handmade wooden cradle for the baby. I want this baby to sleep with us for a long time. But even if we never use the cradle, except as a planter or to hold dolls, it's beautiful.

Martie just called from Ohio. She's coming to visit next week. I'm *so* excited. The weather is perfect. And I feel gorgeous!

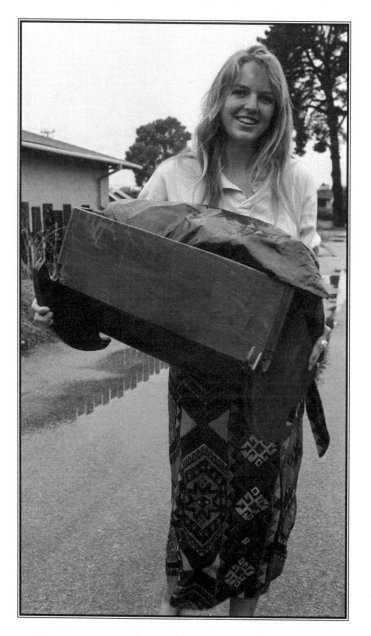

Thank God Martie's here. I need my women friends around me right now. Today we went swimming naked in the ocean. I felt so free! We've been talking about everything, and laughing and playing like kids again. Martie leaves Sunday. God, I wish she could be here for the birth. She says she really wants to. But she can't take that much time off work.

Why can't I just stop working now and do what I really want to do? I'd like to garden and take long walks and bake bread and read, and just *be*. Isn't that enough?

I've begun taking prenatal vitamins with folic acid. My doctor thinks every woman should do it, and her reasons made sense. But I don't know about the tests she wants. I've been reading everything I can about them. I want to be careful about everything that I do—or let anyone else do—to my body now. I don't want to take any risks. And I can't automatically take what others say is best for me or the baby, even if they're "experts." *I'm* the one who has to choose. A lot of people I've talked to seem to think that good prenatal care means getting all the tests. What did they do before they had them?

She wanted to do something called chorionic villi sampling, or at least an amniocentesis, and I didn't feel right about it. Letting them go inside my womb to take cells. It's to see if the baby will have some rare abnormalities. Only they can do it earlier than with amniocentesis. Nowadays, a lot of doctors want to do CVS on everyone. But Jay and I've decided no. I've been reading about the risks of all these tests. We talked about whether we'd have an abortion if the baby was seriously abnormal. I can imagine a situation when I might, but something in me shouted "no!" Not for this baby. Since I decided I wouldn't, no matter what the tests might show, there's no reason to do them.

Mom and I talked about it. I feel like I'm having to protect me *and* this baby. Other women I know think it's all great, especially ultrasound—because they get to take home a picture or even a video of the baby inside the womb. A lot of husbands love it, because it's a machine thing. And also, everyone wants to know the baby's sex ahead of time. We don't. I want some mystery. It's all a big mystery, anyway. Isn't it?

I'm feeling uncomfortable about my doctor. I can tell she doesn't like it when I ask too many questions and don't automatically take her answers as "The Answer."

I've decided the only kind of test I'll allow, unless we suspect there's something wrong, is on my blood or urine. The women I know who allow all these other tests to be done seem a lot more anxious, especially while they wait for the results. It seems like the more tests women have the more uptight their doctors are, and the more anxious *they* are. I don't want to end up being called "high risk." My doctor is acting like, if I let her do all these things, she can guarantee me a perfect baby. Mom reminded me that *nobody* can guarantee that. I think

she's right. I'm glad she and Jay support me in this. Everything's so complicated. I don't want it to be so complicated. I'm healthy and I'm just having a baby!

I'm beginning to wish I'd gone to a midwife. Martie says it's not too late, that I should think about changing. I don't know; it's hard to think about changing now. I want *something* to be stable.

Sitting in the warm sun in the back yard this afternoon, I could feel my anxieties melting away. Don't doctors think about the impact their attitude and choice of words can have on a person?

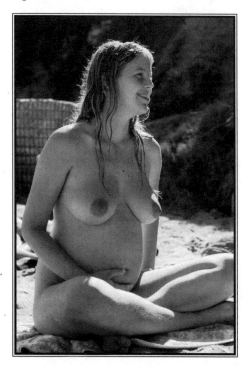

The sky was so clear last night and the stars really stood out. I didn't want to fall asleep. I just kept thinking about this baby and what my life will be like in a few months. And imagining all the other women, all over the world, who are pregnant right now. How many of us are thinking and feeling the same things?

Even though I hardly slept, today I feel full of energy. Now that it's daylight savings time, I can get outdoors after work and it's still daylight after dinner.

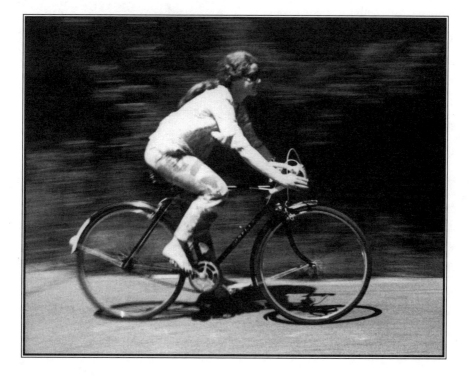

Today I rode my bike for a bit. At first I was a little wobbly and felt off-balance. My belly is getting pretty big. But it was wonderful.

I think I'm a pretty good place for a baby to grow in.

I like to look in the mirror when no one is around and scrutinize the person I see there. I make odd faces and laugh at myself. I bet this baby likes it when I laugh.

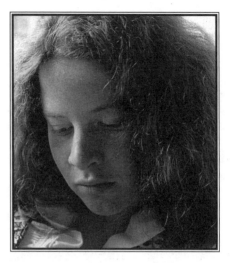

I overheard a woman at my prenatal visit telling another that she hates being pregnant. She said she feels like there's a tumor growing inside her, and that it makes her feel totally out of control, like her body's not hers anymore. I couldn't stop listening. I've never felt any of those things. I felt sad for her.

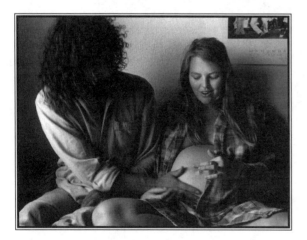

I was talking to a woman at work today about breastfeeding and my plans for after the baby comes. She said she couldn't wait to get rid of all the extra weight after birth. She didn't breastfeed, and immediately went on a diet to lose the weight she'd gained, and went back to Jazzercise classes three weeks after the birth. I kept thinking, what did her baby feel?

I've been obsessing about the birth the past couple days. Finally, I called Mom. I've been looking at some pictures she just sent me of her pregnancy with me, trying to imagine what it was like.

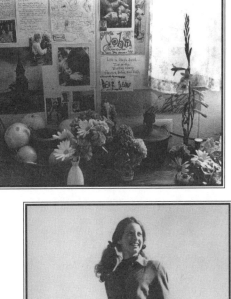

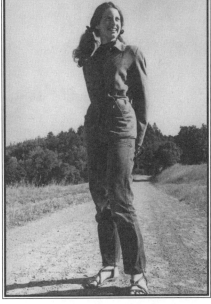

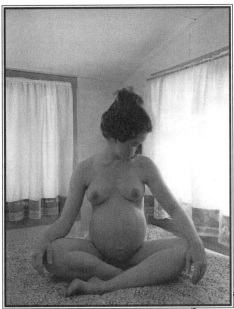

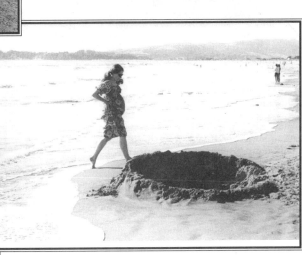

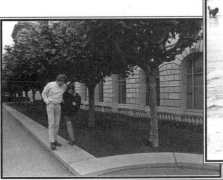

I needed to talk about this birth. I'm thinking I'd be better off having a home birth or going to a birth center. She's all for it. And I think she's hoping I'll ask her to come be with me for the birth. I'd like to have her with me. But I'm not sure. I might not feel like I could really be myself if anyone but Jay's there. Sometimes I don't even want him there.

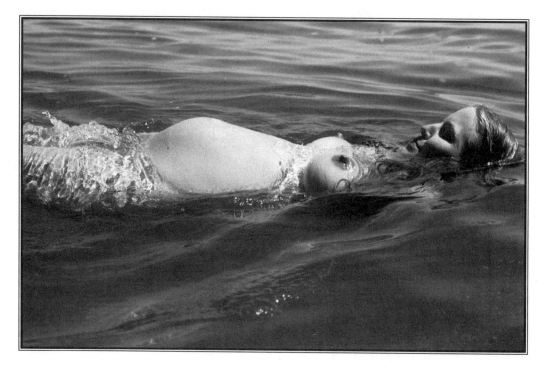

I imagine myself walking off to some secluded stream and having the baby all by myself by the water. A couple nights ago I dreamed I had the baby in the ocean, where it was warm and clear turquoise blue. The baby slipped out and began swimming with me.

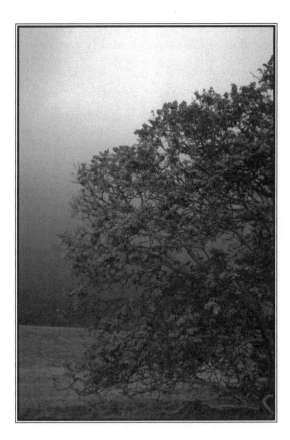

I wonder if there is a birth center around here or anyone who does home births. Jay and I were talking about it last night. He doesn't like the idea of any place but a hospital, but I think he'll go along with what I want. It just might take some time. First, *I* have to know what *I* want.

I've been pissed off a lot the last few days. It's about work. I talked to the baby and told her it's not her fault and I'm not angry at her.

I wonder, are you a girl? I talk about you as if you are, all the time now. I'd like to have a daughter, but either way, I'll be happy.

When I get upset, it helps me to go outside and find a tree to lean my back against. I like to lie on my back in the sun and let it warm my belly. The days still start out cool, but it's almost hot by noon.

Jay and I have been looking at apartments every chance we get. Nothing in our price range is decent. We have to be out of here in three months. I don't want to wait that long. I need to be in our home before this birth.

I'm finding out just how differently Jay and I look at some important things. I never realized it before. For example, in his family kids got spanked, and he says he believes spanking is okay sometimes. He says, "I turned out okay, didn't I?" I told him that's not the point. Hitting a kid just teaches that hitting is okay and that bigger people get to hit smaller people. At least we agreed that we better start doing some talking about our ideas about parenting.

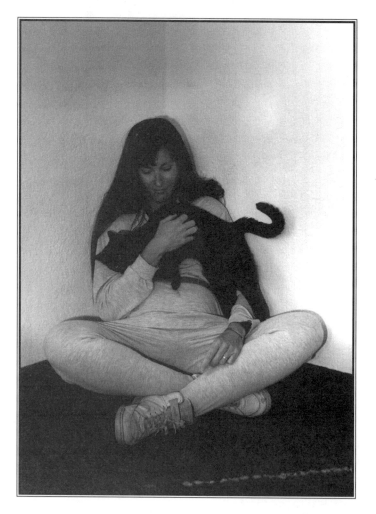

I'm going to get some books. I wish we'd had some courses in high school on how to be a good parent and what kids really need from adults.

Yesterday I made a list of all the things—especially all the bills—I'd have to handle by myself if I end up on my own with this baby. It's not at all what I want, but I better face the possibility. I guess that's one of the givens about being pregnant. It's different for a man.

It makes me feel better to have a picture of everything I'd need and what I'd have to do, instead of just worrying. Now I know how much I'd need to earn for the baby and me. I've made a plan, just in case. I told Mom. She understands. She said she thinks every woman needs to do that, just to know she *can* survive on her own if she has to.

I've been hearing about how many fathers don't pay any child support. I know Jay would not be one of them, but he doesn't earn much. I know I do not want to try to be a superwoman, like Mom says Grandma was. It's not good for kids.

I know one thing. I wouldn't live alone as a single parent. I'd find a place with at least one other single parent and maybe some other adults who'd love to be around my child. It would be less expensive that way, but also better for me and the baby. I'm not such a patient person. I know I would need help.

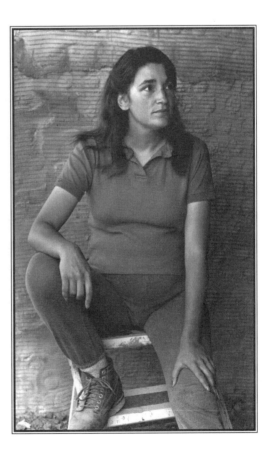

My doctor is pushing me to have a sonogram. Now she's saying she wants to do it to make sure my placenta isn't lying too low and covering the cervix, because that would mean problems and a cesarean.

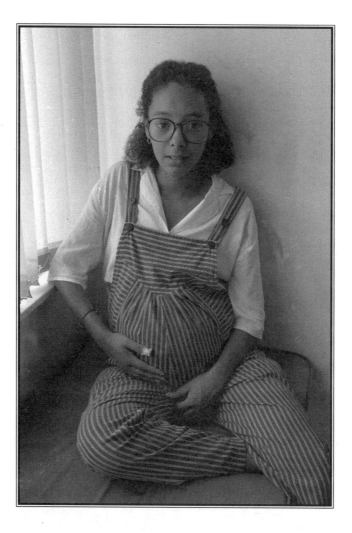

Every time I leave her office I am more worried than when I go in. I'm really thinking about changing to someone else. But who? And it's getting so far along. Next week I'll be six months.

I just realized, *everyone* used to be born at home. I read that women didn't start going to hospitals for birth—except very poor women who had no place decent to live or give birth—until World War I. That was when doctors took control of birth in this country. They tried to turn women away from going to midwives and to put midwives out of business. It was a real smear campaign, from what I've been reading. And midwives are still being harassed or prosecuted for doing home births—even certified nurse-midwives. It's hard to believe that it's only since 1945 that most women have gone to the hospital, yet now it's ninety-nine percent hospital birth! I think about all the women through history who've done it without doctors and hospitals or drugs for pain.

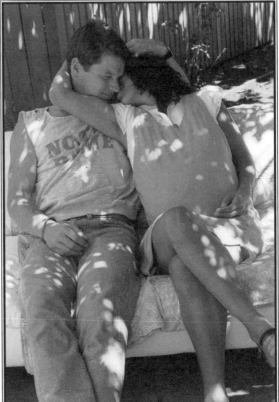

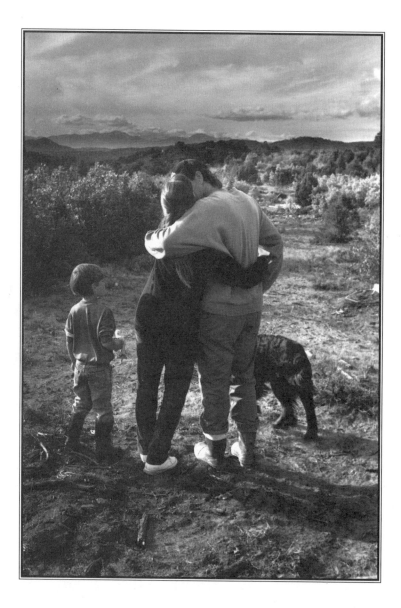

Things have been much better between us this week. I wonder if part of it is that I really looked at what life would be like on my own. I've been feeling less vulnerable. I don't think I've been putting so much on Jay these days.

We're more playful again. We made love last night and I felt closer to Jay than I have in weeks. I needed that so much. I love being pregnant now. It's all the other things I worry about, like where we're going to live and what labor will be like, that sometimes make it hard. I'm sorry, baby, it's not about you. I'm glad you're here.

Jay and I've been talking about where you should be born, Baby. He's nervous about a home birth. I wonder what *his* birth was like? He doesn't have any idea. I suggested he ask his mom. I'm sure that the way we are born makes a big difference about how we feel about the world from then on. Whether our mothers are given drugs, whether we're pulled out or allowed to come out on our own, in our own time, whether we get to be with our mother after birth or are put in a nursery, whether we are held and loved when we cry.

There's so much to think about. The nurse practitioner says my doctor won't even consider doing a home birth. I'd better get some books, do some more reading and talk to more people. This a big decision.

No wonder my mother was so afraid of birth. I just found out what birth was like for her mother. At least it hasn't been kept secret. Great-Grandma Brady—her maiden name was Sulnitzer—was born in Russia and her parents brought her to this country when she a just a child. She was born deaf and grew to be only 4'8" tall. Her doctor told her when she was pregnant with Grandma Davis that she was as strong as an ox and wouldn't have any problem in birth. So, why did she go to the hospital? Mom said it was because it was war-time and there were no doctors doing home birth and very few midwives left, because there had been a campaign to eliminate midwives and put everyone in the hospital for birth.

Great-Grandma told the story that a nurse put her in bed and locked her in the room and left her alone for the entire labor. She said she knew nothing about birth. Her mother had told her nothing! Neither had the doctor. So with each contraction she thought she was dying. Then, when the baby was about to come out, she was knocked unconscious with general anesthesia and missed the whole thing. Grandma was kept in the nursery for several days. Great-Grandma said she never wanted any more children, but since her husband was Catholic, she did get pregnant again and had my great-aunt. She said both her births were so awful she decided she'd never have another, no matter what. Abortion was illegal then, but she told Mom she aborted herself every time she got pregnant, with quinine, and coat hangers. She could have died!

Now that I think about it, it doesn't seem right to have to go to a hospital for a birth unless there's a real problem. Hospitals are for sick people. I'm not sick!

It seems like almost all of the women I've talked to or hear about who gave birth in a hospital had a lot of things done to them they didn't even want: drugs, electronic monitors, IV drips, episiotomy. And so many women are having cesareans. They talk more about the things done to them, all the medical procedures, than the labor or the birth. Everyone wants to tell me their horror story, how they—or the baby—wouldn't have made it if it weren't for the hospital and the doctor. I don't believe it. There's got to be another side to it. But it's enough to make me scared.

Well, Baby, I'm going to change doctors. Yesterday my doctor got on me about gaining too much; she said the birth could be much harder if I gained more than 30 pounds. She's been good-natured up till now, but I opened up the subject of home birth and got a lecture. She said she couldn't imagine why I'd want to put myself—not to mention you, Baby—in jeopardy. I could hardly find any words to answer her, I was so stunned. I felt ashamed, like a little kid in school. But I did manage to ask if she'd ever been to a home birth or a birth in a birth center. She hasn't! So how does she know whether what she believes is true? After I left I got mad.

I took a long walk alone today. Jay and I have been taking more walks, too. But today was extra special. There were hardly any cars, and I found a path in the park that I hadn't taken before. I just lay down on my back and watched the clouds. Several hawks soared over my head, playing in the updraft. I didn't feel lonely. I needed to be alone, I have a lot on my mind.

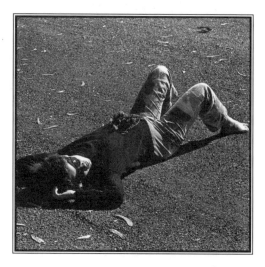

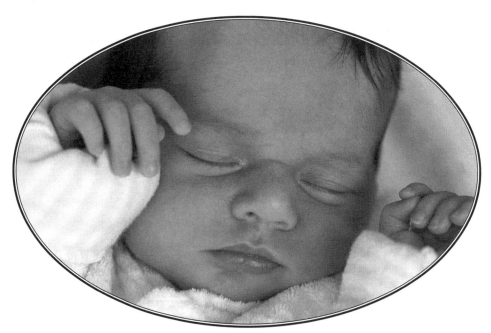

When I'm sleeping, are you awake, Baby? Do you have dreams? What are you dreaming? Now you're part of me. You *are* me in some ways, but you're also *you*. I wish I didn't have to wait all these next months just to see who you are.

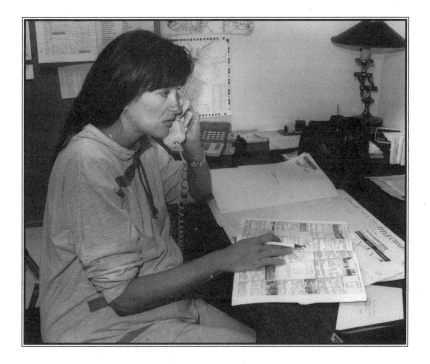

Sometimes I need reminders to take it easy, not to try so hard, not to keep so busy. And not to try to be someone I'm not. This baby needs me to be *me*, to know what *I* want, to take care of myself, and be as calm as I can. I know you're aware of what I'm doing and feeling, Baby. Please be patient with me. I'm doing my best.

I love taking baths. And today I had a massage! I found an ad in the health food store for a woman who specializes in massage for pregnant women. She was great. I felt like I was on a cloud, floating in warm sunshine. I can't believe I haven't treated myself to this before. I want Jay and I to learn how to massage each other.

Well, Baby, today I sent a letter to my doctor saying I'm not coming back. I couldn't do it face-to-face. I gave my reasons. I decided she should have feedback from patients about her attitude. It may not do any good, but it may. I want doctors to know that some women don't appreciate being talked to as if they are ignorant. I would never do anything purposely that I thought might hurt you, Baby.

I want us to have the best possible birth. Jay and I have to talk tonight. I don't care how tired he is. He may not agree with what I want, but I'm the one carrying you inside me. I'm the one who has to go through labor. I'm the one who feels scared of the pain. And *I'm* the one who has to feel right about the birth. Does that sound irresponsible?

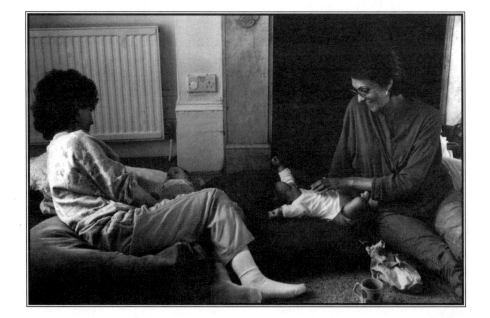

Jay supported me in not going back to my doctor. I shouldn't have been surprised. He's really been paying attention to my desires lately, and he's growing more and more excited about being a papa. But he's nervous about having a home birth. I would go to a birth center, but I've already found out there isn't one around here. I've been hearing stories that the hospital that claims to have the most modern birthing unit has just as high an epidural anesthesia rate, just as high a cesarean rate, and just as many babies ending up in the intensive care nursery as the other hospitals. They aren't really in support of natural childbirth. There are too many rules.

I wish Jay could *really* feel what it's like to carry this baby. He tries. But he can't. I want him to know how much I think about what's best for the baby. Sometimes I wish I lived in a village where all the women gathered around the fire each night to share their stories, and where all the women helped each other in birth.

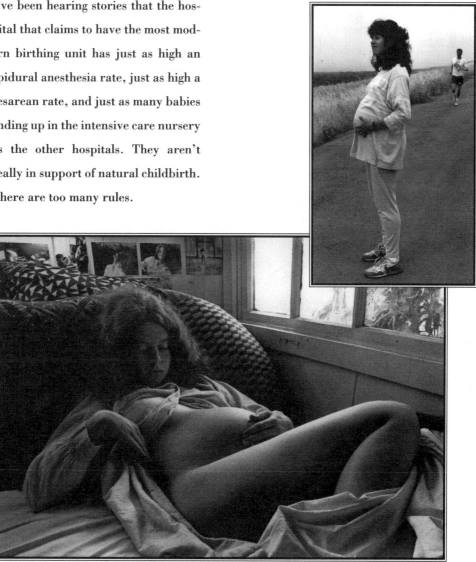

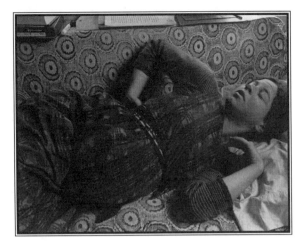

I've been having homeless dreams. What if we can't find a place before the baby comes? We found one apartment we like and can afford—barely—but it won't be available for two months. That's too long. I think we may have to move in with friends for a couple of weeks. Thank God we have friends who've offered!

I want a midwife.

I've been reading about what makes midwives different from doctors, and I want to find a midwife. I feel guilty for telling my doctor I'm not coming back. Like I'm supposed to be a good girl. I know it's not my job, but I feel like I should somehow protect *her* from my feelings. Whose birth *is* this, anyway?

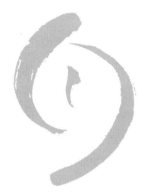

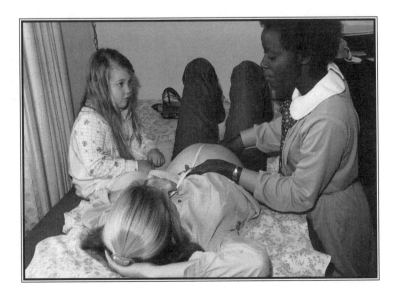

I can't believe how vulnerable I feel these days around the issue of a place to live. I can't imagine what a woman must go through who is homeless and pregnant.

I've never felt really beautiful, but I've liked my face and I've always liked my hands, my feet and my breasts. Now my body and my face are becoming so filled out, I hardly look like the me I know. Sometimes I don't recognize myself when I catch my reflection. Who is that person? You're making me change, Baby. Who will I be by the time you arrive?

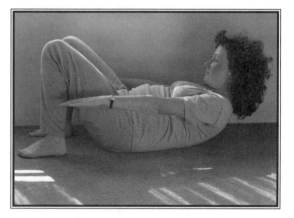

Well, we've decided. Jay told his parents we are going to have a home birth, unless something happens and we need the hospital. Today he's really been acting nervous, because both his parents got on the phone and they tried to convince him that you, or both of us—could die. He's feeling so responsible and not in control. I don't feel in control, either. All these changes inside me. But I can't let other people make decisions for us, Baby. I'm going to see if there's a class for people planning a home birth, so we can be around some other people wanting what we want.

Somewhere, deep inside I must know what is right for me and right for you, Baby. My body *must* know how to give birth. Women have been doing it for eons, and having healthy babies.

I called the doctor's office today, since I got no answer from my letter. The receptionist said the doctor was too busy to call me back today. She also said I couldn't have my records back, that I have to have my next physician order them. They're *my* records. Why would she assume I'm going to another doctor?! In my letter I even said I'd decided to see a midwife. I got angry at her, but I apologized. It's not her fault. I just wish women would support each other.

I just found out that some people tried to open a birth center not far from one of the hospitals, half an hour from here. But no obstetricians would do births there *or* back up midwives doing births there. No insurance company would insure it, and this state won't allow a birth center to open without insurance. Democracy in action! I don't want to be political right now. I just want to be pregnant! I don't want to fight to get what I want for us. I'm just having a baby. Why does it have to be so complicated?

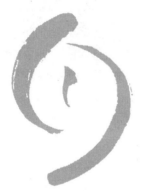

My doctor never did call me back or write. I've given it too much energy. I'm not going to give it any more, Baby. You need my attention. You need me to be good to myself and as happy as I can be.

I'm almost certain you're a girl! Sometimes at night before we go to sleep Jay plays with you, plays games on my belly, trying to communicate with you. Do you know that? I know you can hear his voice. He loves you very much. I've been playing some special music all week, because I just found out that you can hear inside your womb home. It's very peaceful music. I think I'll put together some tapes just for the birth—to help me stay calm, but also for you.

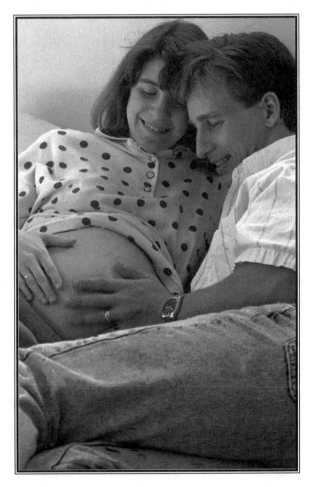

It's perfect how things work out! I should trust more. When I think of *all the time* I've spent worrying. Today I met a woman in the store with a three-month-old baby who had a home birth. She said she's so glad she did it that way, and she told me the name of her midwife.

I just *had* to ask her about the pain. She said it hurt like hell when labor really got going, that nothing had prepared her for what contractions really felt like. But, she said, having her husband with her, and two of her best friends, plus her midwife and an assistant there, was the support she needed. She said, "It was worth *every* bit of the pain, just to be totally conscious and feeling everything." She even felt her baby slip out of her body.

She said, because she took no drugs, he was very alert. "He came out with his eyes open and looked right up at me even while his legs were still inside! When he was in my arms, he looked right into everyone's eyes, took it all in. He never did cry."

"I felt like a Goddess—and I'm still feeling high from it." Her baby's so beautiful. She gave me her phone number so we could talk some more. I couldn't wait to tell Jay.

I called the midwife. Her name is Roxanne. She called me back after dinner and we talked for twenty minutes. She wants to meet with me on Friday at the end of her day. She said we'll talk about what I'm looking for and see if we might work out well together. And she doesn't charge anything for that visit! I'm not sure our insurance will pay for a midwife, I have to talk to the insurance company. I've already told Jay if it won't, we'll have to borrow the money, because that's not a good enough reason to change my mind. One more thing to think about, when all I want to do is be pregnant. But at last I feel like things are falling into place for us, Baby.

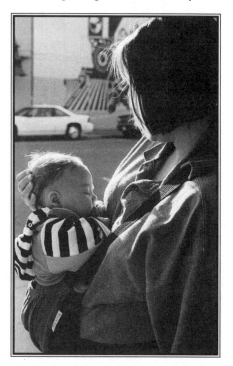

I've never loved a dawning as
much as today.

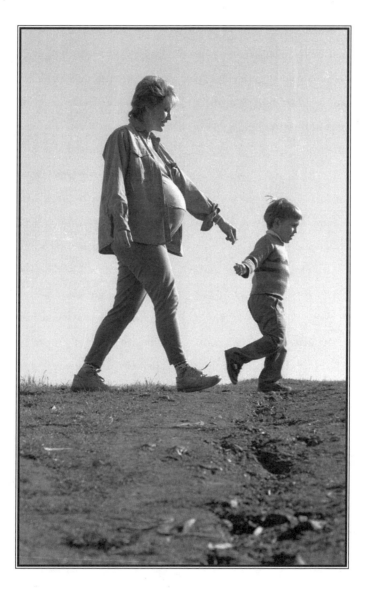

Jay took time off work to go to see Roxanne with me. We couldn't believe how comfortable we felt. She treated us like equals, took all of our concerns seriously, and she answered every question we asked. She says that since I'm in good health, there's no reason to believe I'll have problems, so she can take me for a home birth! Mostly it was the gut feeling I had that she's the one I want to be with me. Jay said he felt it too.

Roxanne can't do births at any hospital around here—even though she's legal and licensed.

The hospitals still won't give midwives privileges. Roxanne was told she "might" get them if she works for a doctor, but she said she doesn't want to work for a hospital or a doctor. She likes independence, even if it does mean she has no formal backup now. She does have one obstetrician she refers clients to when she has questions. There's only one in the whole county who'll see midwives' clients! And if that OB is out of town, she said we'd have to take pot luck if we needed doctor backup at the hospital. I didn't realize how much of a political issue birth is today.

Anyway, if you or I needed to be in the hospital, Baby, Roxanne says she'd go with us. But she couldn't be "in charge." That's not likely to happen anyway, because we're healthy, you and I. Roxanne works with an assistant, an apprentice midwife, who goes to all the home births with her. She says it's so she has an extra pair of hands in case of a problem, but also because she believes every midwife should train others to pass along the knowledge, since a lot of what midwives do is so different from what doctors or nurses are taught. Her transfer rate to the hospital is just ten percent, and that is because she's cautious. Her cesarean rate is less than five per cent. It all makes me feel good.

Roxanne says she *loves* doing births in women's own homes. She considers it a privilege to be invited into a woman's home to be with her in birth, and that it's where she sees women come into their real strength during labor. I'm so glad I found her. I'll bet you're glad too, baby!

With enough support, I think I can go through labor on my own, without drugs.

I asked Roxanne to do a pelvic exam on me because my doctor had said my pelvis was a little small. Normally it's not something she would do on a first visit. She said my pelvis is a perfect size, even if I have a pretty big baby. I said, "I bet you tell that to everyone!" And she said, "Yes, I do."

"I've found it helps labor go normally if I give a woman a positive feeling about her pelvis." She said there's no point in putting fear into a woman about her pelvic dimensions, since pelvises expand in labor—especially if the woman is squatting for the birth—and that a baby's head is made to mould to the shape of its mother's pelvis. I didn't know this, but she said it's exceedingly rare for a baby not to be able to fit through its own mother's pelvic bones, unless the baby is in an unusual position. When it has happened, she's found the cause was always malpresentation, the baby lying in a slightly unusual way. Doctors talk about CPD—the baby's head being too big for the mother's pelvis. But she said midwives hardly ever see CPD, even when the mother is petite and the father very large. Hearing this made Jay feel better, too.

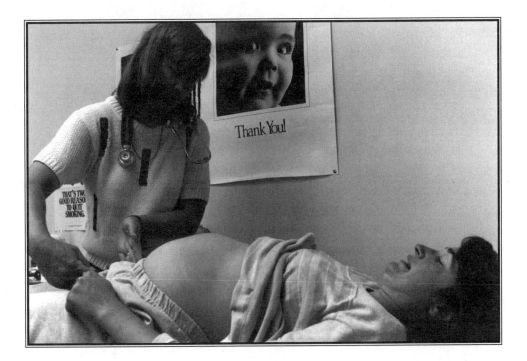

I feel so good! I just ran five
blocks and I feel like telling the whole
world I'm going to be a mother!

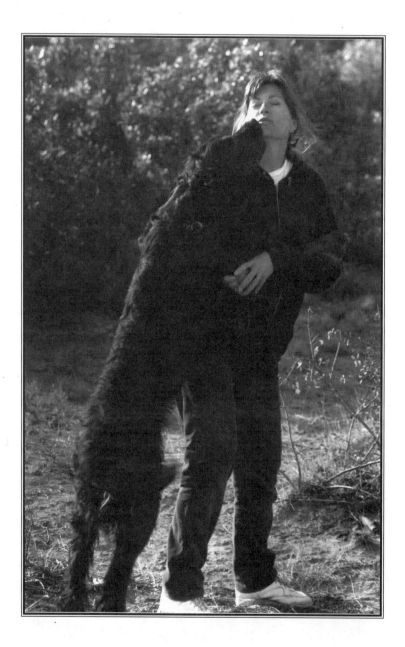

Jay and I've been doing some more reading about home birth and the risks. So many people we know talk about "high-risk" hospitals as if they're the safest place to birth. But not according to what I've been reading. I feel like I'm becoming an expert. Roxanne reminded me that a birthing woman *is* an authority. Her body knows what to do and should be trusted. Planned home births with a skilled attendant are apparently just as safe for a mother and baby as being in the most highly equipped hospital. That's not talking about unplanned home births—births that just happen at home without anyone planning it that way—because the baby comes too fast for the women to go anywhere. Those births usually happen without any skilled attendant. According to

what I just read, home births or birth centers are actually safer than hospital births for healthy women, because there's so much unnecessary intervention done in hospitals, and medical intervention makes birth more risky. Especially if it means the baby ends up in an intensive care nursery when it doesn't have any real need to be there—"just in case." Why doesn't anybody talk about this?

All the women I know who had cesareans, or whose babies ended up in intensive care, act as if it was one big emergency. They seem so afraid of birth, so sure they—or the baby—needed everything that was done. It's so different being around a woman who's had a good and normal birth, especially a birth center or home birth. I got together with Jane yesterday—the woman I met at the grocery store who had a home birth. Her baby is so lovely—and it was great being with someone who has good things to say about birth. I just drank it all in. Her attitude is so different from most of the women I know. I asked her, "How did you get so strong?" She said she wasn't always this way, she had a lot of fears from how she was raised. She says the birth has made her much more confident in herself.

It's a miracle! All this happening inside me. Today after work I went and sat with my back up against the trunk of my favorite tree down at the park. I always feel good by that tree. I really feel your spirit, Baby. We're friends. I'm getting to know you more and more. It's going to feel so good to look into your face and hold you in my arms. Soon.

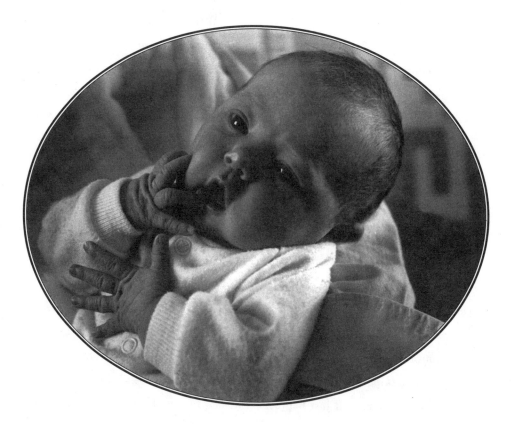

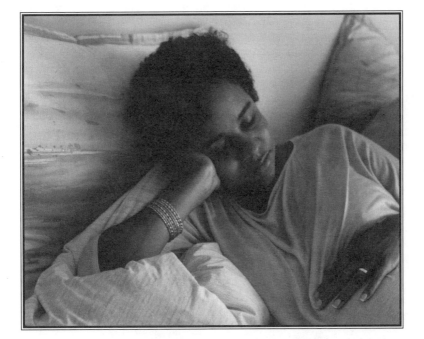

Today, at my visit, Roxanne asked me about my feelings about my body, and we got talking about sex. I told her, ever since I became pregnant I've been getting more and more pleasure from sex and that I'm feeling sensual. I told her how uptight I used to be sexually. She gave me some simple things I can do to practice letting go in lovemaking, that will help me give in to contractions in labor.

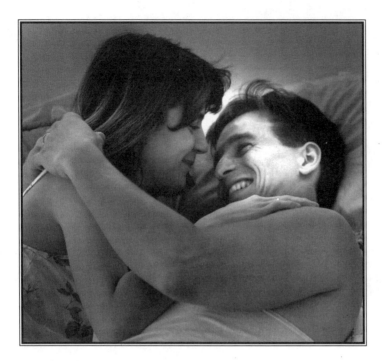

My old tightness seems to be losing its hold on me. Sometimes Jay is worried about hurting the baby when we make love. But mostly he's glad I'm freer and enjoying myself more. *Me* too.

I heard from a woman who was in the Peace Corps about a tribe in Africa. They have a story they pass down from woman to woman to inspire a woman who is about to give birth. The woman in labor must cross a shallow but rushing river, and the only way she can get to the other side is by walking on a very long, slippery log that stretches across the river. She has to keep her balance or she'll fall into the rushing water. But she is told, "you will not be alone on your crossing." All the women of her village go with her, walking through the rushing water, holding her steady, until she is safe on the other shore. I like that image. Of a woman having to do it on her own, yet not being alone.

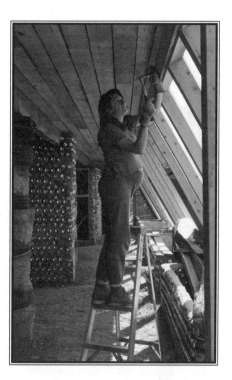

What will labor be like? What if I'm one of those women who takes forever to dilate? Can I be patient? Will I have the endurance? Will I be a baby about the pain and ask for drugs?

I'm going to the bookstore and library and see if I can find any books of stories about birth in other cultures and see what women in other places do, especially if labor is long.

I've been wanting to make love often for the past few weeks. Now that Jay and I are really close, it just brings us that much closer. He's very gentle, and we've become more creative, since my belly is getting so big. I can't believe how wonderful our sex life is. I get so aroused these days. I've read that some women don't feel at all sexy in pregnancy. I'm glad I'm not one.

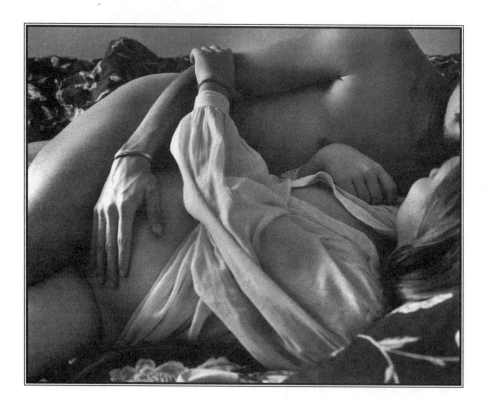

How many times will it take before I learn that things *do* work out without my trying to control everything? Today we found a place we both liked and can afford. I think the landlord's going to give it to us. It's a little small, but very light, and we decided we'd rather pay less and be less stressed, especially since I'm not going back to work until you're at least nine months, Baby. A baby's only a baby for a short time.

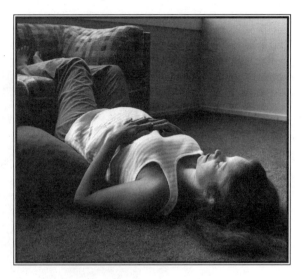

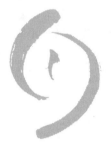

Jay began talking about how he'd like to take time off after you come, Baby, and be a *real* parent. He doesn't want to miss out on your first months. He's going to see what he can do. It's hard, because there's no support for fathers at his job. He's been taking on extra work, even on weekends, so we can put some money aside. I miss him when he's working so hard. There's none of him left for us, he's so tired. But I really appreciate it, too. He's doing it all for us.

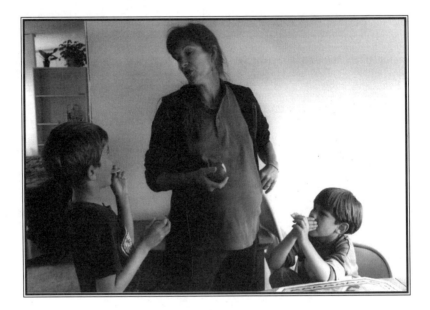

My mom offered to help us out in the first months, and I think Jay's parents might too. Jay's too proud to ask, but maybe they'll bring it up when he talks to them about what our plans are. They're all glad that we're not going to put this baby in day care when its young. Boy, are we lucky to have family who care.

Waiting...

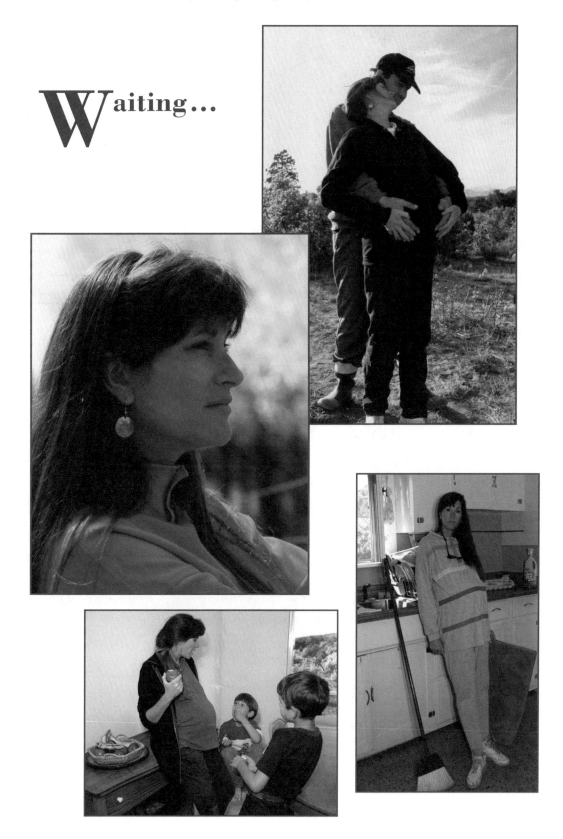

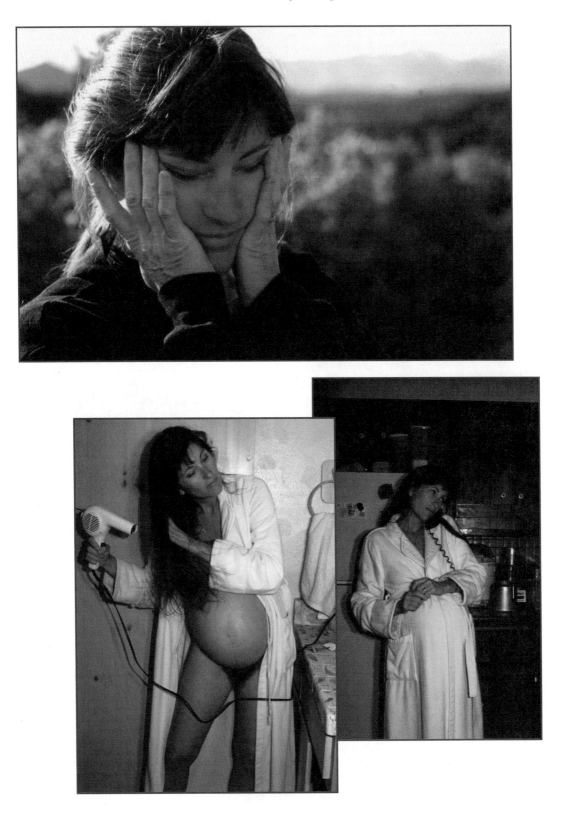

Until...

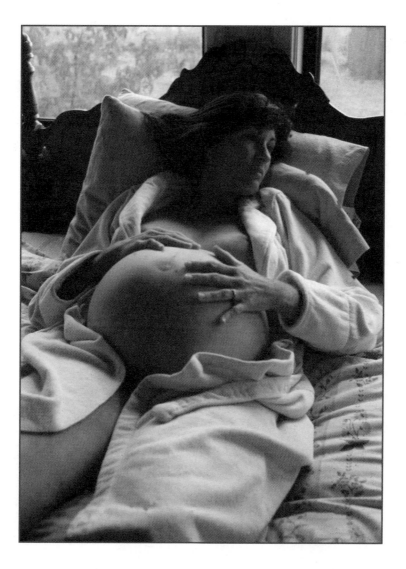

Forty weeks

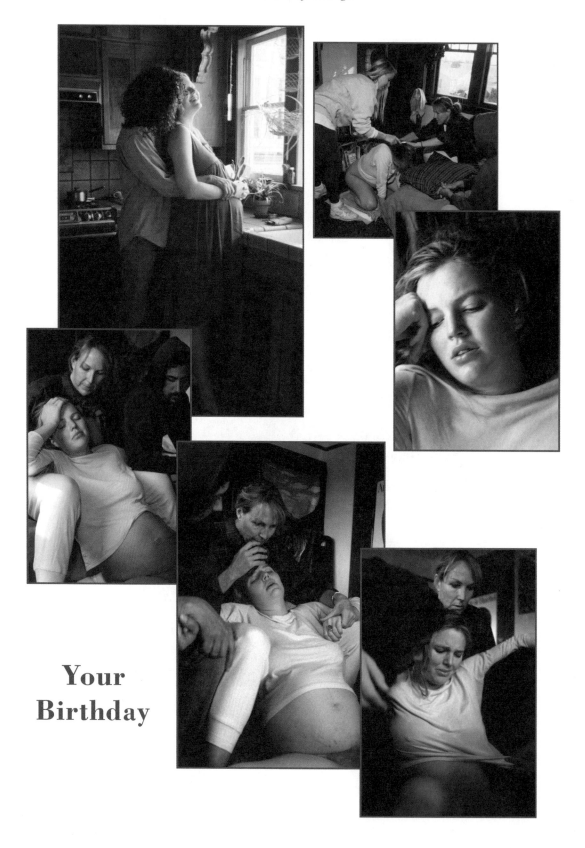

Your
Birthday

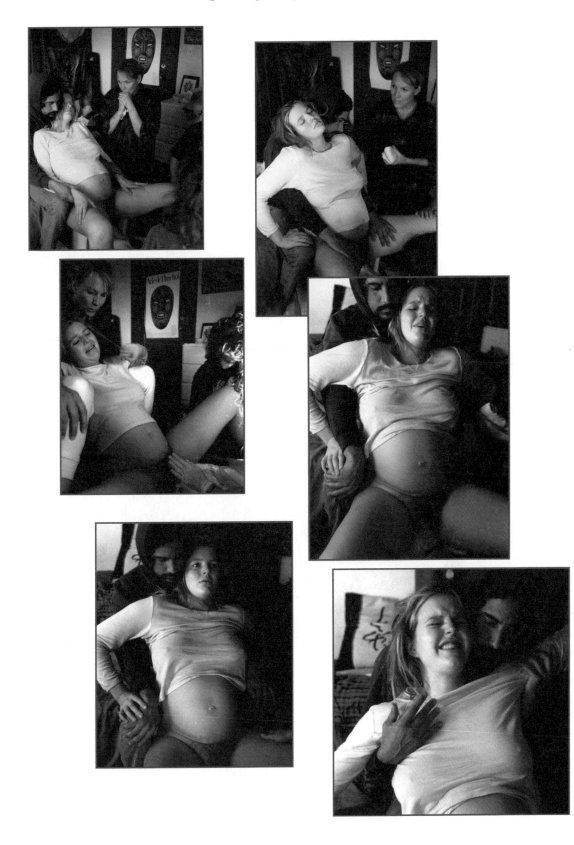

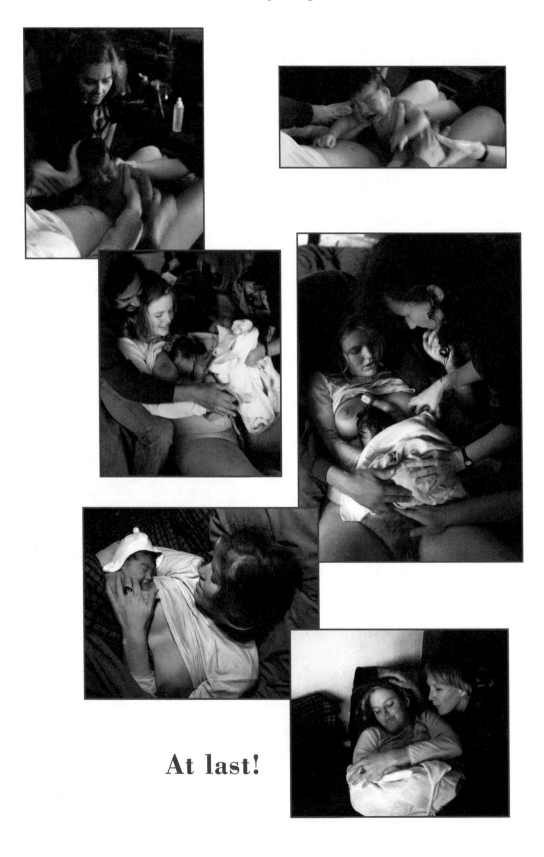

At last!

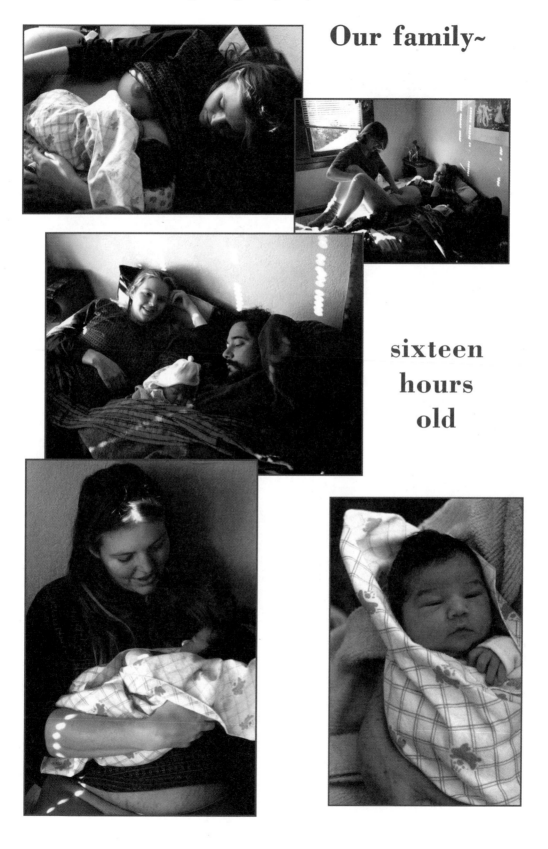

Our family~

**sixteen
hours
old**

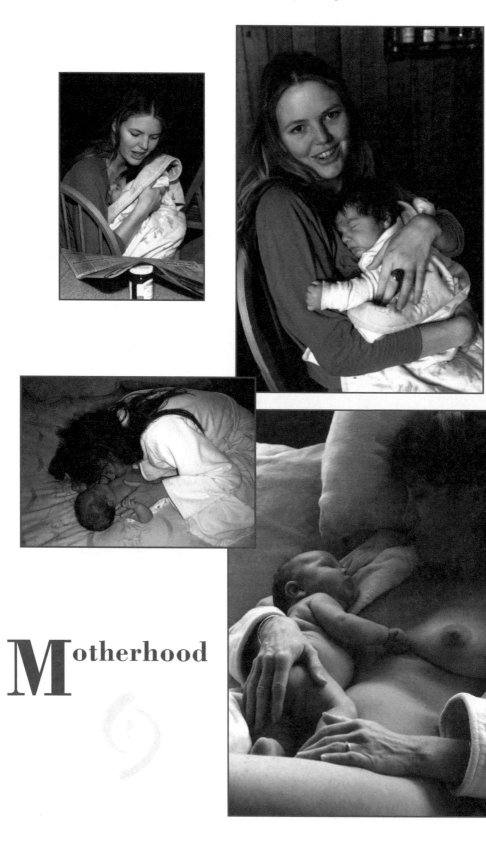

Motherhood

I've been making plans for our new apartment—colors and ideas for furnishings. The bedroom and kitchen have lots of morning light. I can wake up to the sun instead of an alarm. We can lie in bed with you, Baby, and watch the sunrise.

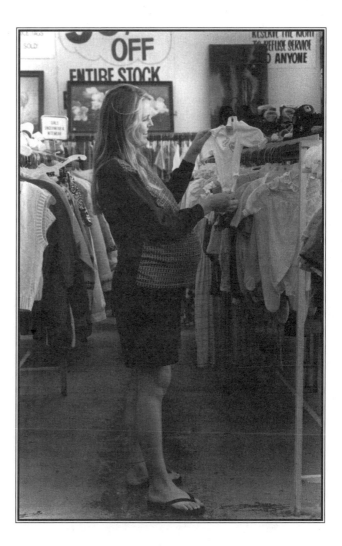

This weekend we start packing up. I'm getting excited. It feels right. Getting a new home for your arrival.

I've been dreaming a lot lately. In color too.

Had a strange dream last night: baby animals popping up in all sorts of unexpected places. I opened my bureau drawer and found six tiny, gray, striped kittens. But the mama wasn't there.

My friend said she dreamed at the end of pregnancy that her baby came out and asked for nachos. She works in a Mexican restaurant.

Last night I dreamed you were falling off a mountain, Baby. We were in a car, and I couldn't catch hold of you in time. It was horrible! I guess I'm really beginning to feel like a mother. When Jay drives us somewhere—and he's always been a careful driver—I find myself holding my belly to protect you.

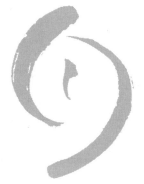

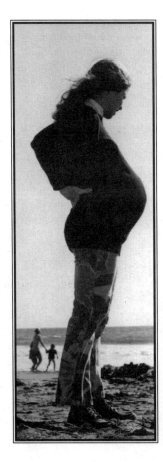

Last week Carolyn came to visit—
and to help me pack. She brought a
wooden stethoscope with her that she
borrowed from someone who just
came back from Holland. It's made
from a light colored, lightweight wood
and is shaped like the kind of ear
trumpets I've seen pictures of people
using before hearing aids were
invented. She said midwives—and
even some doctors—still use these in
Holland to listen to the baby's heart. I
liked it, like the feel of it in my hand.
It's like a piece of sculpture. We tried,
but we couldn't find the riqht spot to
hear your heartbeat, Baby. So we
borrowed a regular stethoscope from
Roxanne. Your heart is so strong.

I went to see a chiropractor
today. My lower back has been hurting a lot. She massaged the area and
then did a very gentle adjustment on
my sacrum. I feel much better.

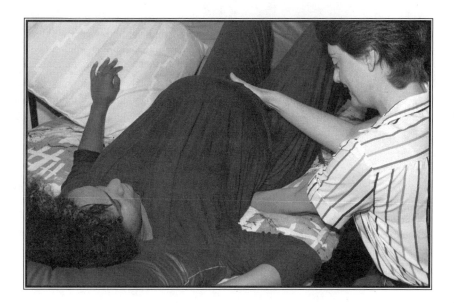

We're having hiccups! My belly is bouncing up and down. They're your hiccups. It's so strange. Where do you end and I begin?

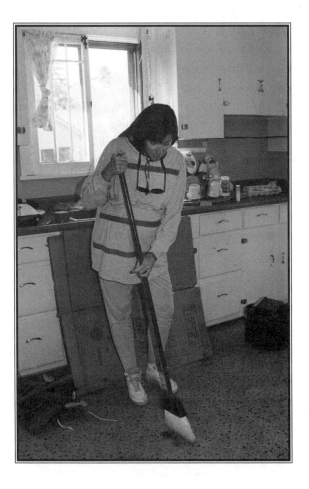

Moving day! I'm so exhausted from packing up. I don't think I could have done it if we waited one more week. Time is zipping by. There's so much to do before you come. I need a little more time.

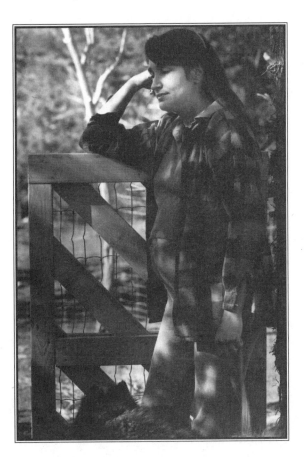

There aren't enough hours in the day. So many things I want to do before you come, baby. Including taking naps, reading long novels. I hear I won't have any time to myself soon. That's such a strange idea. I'm glad I have a little more time just to be me.

How can I possibly be a good enough mother for this baby when I'm so impatient. I better work on controlling my temper!

Roxanne reminded me to take advantage of the time now, before you come, to do the kinds of things I've always wanted to do, and might not be able to do once I'm a mother.

We're here! Our new home. I was so looking forward to it. But then, at breakfast this morning I fell completely to pieces and couldn't stop crying. I don't know what's going on with me. I've really lost it.

I cry over the silliest things.

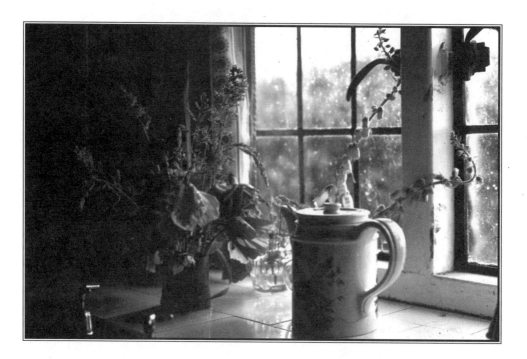

I don't want to go to work. I don't want to leave the apartment—except to sit in the park and look up at the sky. I like to sit and look out the window and let my mind go blank.

Yesterday I unpacked my bike and went for a ride today. I think it will be my last time before you come, Baby. My balance is poor, but I was careful, and it felt good to feel the air against my body.

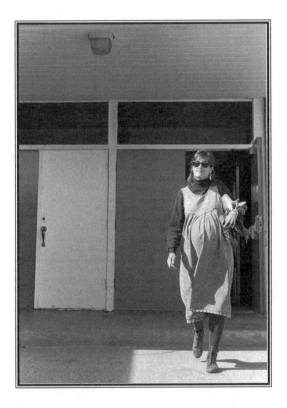

Today I took a backpack and went to the park. I ate both sandwiches before I got there and was hungry an hour later. I've gained 31 pounds already. I feel great!

I've been buzzing around, too busy to sit still. The curtains are up and I've been crocheting a blanket for you, Baby. Jay laughs at me and says I'm half-crazed. He's right.

I love our new home and coming home to it, walking in the door and smelling the special smell. I bought a big flowering plant for the dining room table today. It should bloom all the way until you get here, Baby.

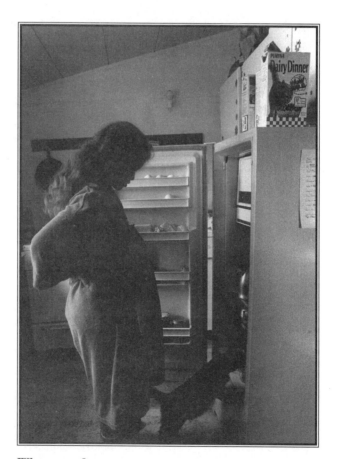

What to eat?

We're going to a series of birth classes that's aimed at people who want to avoid unnecessary cesareans or other intervention, and have natural childbirth. It's a small class, just four couples. Well, three couples and one single woman and a friend of hers who'll be at the birth. I guess there aren't too many people who want a natural birth these days. Almost everyone's going to the free classes they teach at the hospital.

Last night was the first class. At the end our teacher, Faye, asked each of us to find out as much as we could about what our mother's pregnancy with us was like, how she felt about labor, the way we were born, and what our hours after birth and first weeks were like. For instance, was the birth complicated, were there drugs, did we go to the nursery, did our mom breastfeed?

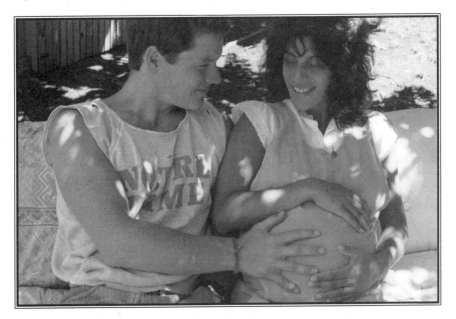

She told us there's evidence that a lot of women follow the pattern of their mother's labor—whether it's short or long. She also talked about what our experiences are in the womb, and how the way we are born leaves indelible impressions on our nervous system and can set up lifelong patterns. I felt good that I already knew that because of what I've been reading. Jay's going to talk to his mom this week about his birth.

I wish I could go to a birth—a *normal* birth—so I can know what it's like. Mom says you never really know till you go through it yourself, because every one is so different. She's right, but still....

Today I talked to a woman I've seen around but have never talked to before. I was standing in front of the deli section spacing out like I do a lot, unable to make up my mind what I wanted—and she came up and told me how great I look pregnant. Then she asked me how my pregnancy has been going. It felt good to be noticed. She told me how much she enjoyed the last months of her pregnancy, said she misses those special feelings of being so alive. I told her I have boundless energy these days, that I've started making homemade bread and making a quilt for the baby and sewing. She smiled and nodded. We walked outside together and stood on the street. I felt very close to her. Yet we didn't even bother to ask each other's name.

Friends keep coming up to me to pat my belly or "talk" to you, Baby. I get more attention now than I ever did before. I feel like the first woman on earth to be pregnant.

Some days I don't want people poking at me. Everyone—even strangers—seem to think it's okay to come up and pat my belly. I'm on display all the time. I have no privacy at all! Sometimes I don't want so much attention from Mom. She's been calling me every few days this week. I need some space!

We're saving up as much money as we can, so I can take at least six whole months off after you're here, Baby. I want to be with you and take care of you. I know a lot of women say they have to go back to work just a few weeks after the birth. I think that's awful, especially when they have to leave their baby with someone else the whole day! I want to be a full-time mom for the first nine months if we can do it. Then I only want to start back to work part time. I'm going to talk to my supervisor.

I may have to quit and look for work I can do at home or a job where I can take you with me, Baby. I've gotten Jay thinking about it too. It's not fair that he can't be with you a lot of the time too, Baby. We're going to work it out, somehow.

Two of the women in my birth class have parents who don't agree with them having a natural birth and who are full of awful warnings. I'm so fortunate. I think I'll call Mom tonight and thank her for all her support.

I know a woman who's only three days past her due date, but her doctor's already talking about inducing labor or having to do a cesarean. Thank God I'm not going to someone like that. Talk about pressure!

The clouds have been just beautiful these past couple of days. And the air is clean because it rained last night.

I love taking my walks now. It's so warm I don't even need a sweater in the evening. And it's still light till mid-evening. I try to walk an hour a day. Our birth teacher says it's a great way to get exercise but also a great way to clear our heads of too much thinking and worrying. She calls it walking meditation and suggests we focus all our attention on just breathing and the feeling of each step. I've been doing that. I've found another woman in the class who wants to take long walks with me a couple times a week before or after dinner.

At class this week we watched six different births. They were all normal but each one had something slightly unusual about them—like a knot in the cord or the cord around the baby's neck, or the baby in posterior position. One was a very long dilation phase. Our teacher talked about the difference between variations on normal and true abnormality in birth.

There's lots of variation in what is normal. That's good to know. I'm getting so much more confidence.

At my prenatal visit I asked Roxanne about the different things that can happen and still let me have a home birth. She said most things that arise in labor that could be a problem—like getting to a certain point in the cervix dilating and then having dilation stop for several hours or more—are self-correcting. That nothing needs to be done, except to make sure the woman is as comfortable as possible and taking as much nourishment—especially liquids—as possible. She said sometimes a labor needs a bit of help, like getting a woman to change positions if the baby's heart tones slow down. Some things do need active intervention. But even then, she said, the intervention isn't necessarily medical. Often it's as simple as getting the woman to drink more and empty her bladder and get up and move around.

She said she's found drugs and artificial hormones are seldom needed. She takes oxygen with her to every birth, in case the baby needs a little extra afterward. And she carries medication in case I bleed too much after the birth. But at home you won't have to have antibiotic ointment in your eyes, Baby, unless I want it. The book I'm reading says that you'll be able to see more clearly in the first hours after birth—because the birth creates a brain growth spurt—than for weeks afterward. And that the distance that a baby sees most clearly is 8-12 inches, which is the distance its eyes are from its mother's eyes when a baby is breast-feeding. Amazing! I don't want anything put in your eyes. Jay's as fascinated as I am with all this. It's like entering a whole new world.

Roxanne told me that most of what I need for a normal labor is having the people around me I trust and get comfort from, my own familiar surroundings, the things I like to eat and drink to keep my body's strength up, and a positive attitude. She also said that the point of having a midwife stay with you once active labor sets in that she can observe you and tell early on if you need something only a doctor or hospital can provide.

She said if we need to go to the hospital there will most likely be enough time to leave without a rush and go in our own car. She's seldom had a real emergency, one that needed calling an ambulance or 911. In those couple of times, she's done first aid until the ambulance arrived. She's not taking any chances. Jay told his parents that, and I think they're feeling a little better about our decision. I'm glad she always takes an assistant with her to births, just to help.

It's not that I want to be ignorant. But I wish people were sensitive to how vulnerable a pregnant woman can feel—at least how vulnerable I feel, and exposed. I take everything anyone says to me right in. Sometimes I should protect myself, because people can be thoughtless.

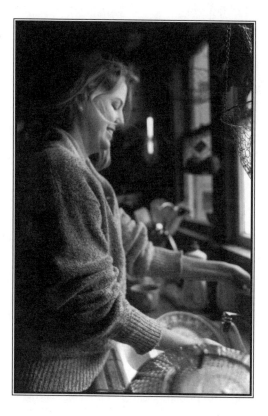

Jay's been trying to get things arranged so he can take time off as soon as you're here, Baby. He wants to be with us. If he has to, he'll take his vacation then. Or unpaid leave. Why isn't taking care of a baby considered important enough for it to be taken into account? You'd think he was asking something awful. There are more important things than work—people. I feel really grateful that Jay's become so committed to being a father.

Oh dear. Roxanne says you're breech, Baby. That you're lying with your butt down toward my pelvis. My due date is eight weeks, and if you stay breech, she says she can't do a home birth with me, because it's a bit higher risk. Damn! Please turn, Baby. It's getting close to when you'll drop down into my pelvis, and then you won't be able to turn.

I'm supposed to get a lot of exercise this week, especially walking, but also stretching and squatting, to see if you'll turn on your own, like a lot of babies do who are breech at the eighth month. If you're still breech next week she wants to try and turn you. She says that most of the time it works. Her partner Kate has had more experience than she at turning breeches, so Kate would do it.

One more surprise. I better learn how to handle surprises, because they keep coming. I sure wish you'd turn. Roxanne told me to find a tuning fork—the kind singers use—and to lie on the floor with my bottom up on a couple of pillows or thick books, and then make the tuning fork ring. She said that sometimes will get a baby to turn, to get away from the vibration of the sound. Please, Baby...

At class we learned that breastfeeding isn't all instinctual. We were all surprised. It's mostly something the mother and baby have to learn by spending time together. I also learned it helps if you have been breastfed yourself and have gotten to watch women breastfeeding as you're growing up. I was breastfed, but Jay wasn't. But my mom said that the first time she ever saw anyone breastfeed a baby, she was in college—and then the woman left the dinner party to do it in the bedroom!

My cousin just had her first baby—a cesarean. I wonder if it was necessary. My aunt said she never dilated. She's not breastfeeding, didn't even want to try. If there's anything she and her baby needed after a cesarean birth and the baby spending time in the nursery, I'd think it would be breastfeeding.

We learned a couple of techniques for focusing attention in labor and staying centered, keeping our attention on our breath. It's to help me ride or float on the pain of the contractions, without panicking. She says it's something we can use all through our lives, whenever we're under a lot of stress or getting overwhelmed with fear or anger. We're supposed to practice. I'm practicing it to get you to turn, Baby. Jay borrowed a tuning fork. I'm going to try that, too.

Jay's been talking at work about what we're learning in birth class. He's been surprised by how much the other guys want to hear about what we're doing. It's so interesting, because a lot of women I run into don't show any interest in natural birth and are really shocked at our planning to do it at home.

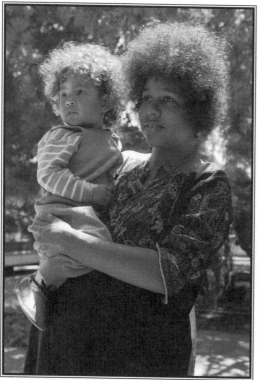

Today Jay took off work and went with me for Kate to turn you, Baby. She was really good. So were you! I like the way her hands felt. It didn't seem to bother you—your heart rate didn't even speed up. But what did it feel like to you? I had heard it would hurt, but it wasn't painful for me.

I lay on my back. First, Kate pushed her fingers down and in, into my pelvis, under you. That made you pop up out of it. It was an intense feeling, and weird, but it wasn't pain. I was watching my belly, and it mounded up like a wave. I got nervous at the feeling—I laugh when I get nervous—so I began to laugh. Then the most *amazing* thing happened. I could see you moving as you turned all the way around! Jay couldn't believe it either.

We went home and took a long walk, like she and Roxanne suggested. Please don't turn back, Baby.

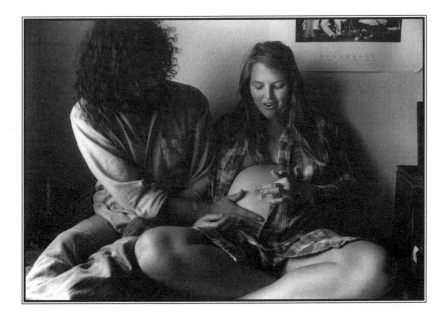

I've been writing in my diary every day. I'm trying to find time for a little meditation and a walk, too. It's easier to just sit down and watch TV after work. But watching TV doesn't make me feel as good. When I sit quietly and write—sometimes I draw—and then sit with my back straight and focus just on my breathing, instead of my thoughts, even if I just do it for five minutes, I notice the difference all evening. It's not easy. When I can, I like to get up earlier and sit before breakfast. It makes the day go better. And sometimes Jay does it with me. Our teacher said the most important thing is becoming a friend to our breath, just being with it, and letting the thoughts come into our mind without following them with our attention. I think I'd like to take a meditation class some day and learn more about it.

I talked to my aunt today and after telling me how worried she is that I'm having a home birth, she said, "Well, let's just hope for a healthy baby." She has so little faith. I really have to be careful about talking to her, or anyone else who is full of fears. It's contagious.

So many of the "what if this and what if that happens" thoughts don't seem to be really a part of me but things that got planted in me somewhere along the way as I grew up. I've been looking at each one to see if it's something I should ask the midwife about or do something about. A lot of my fears don't seem helpful at all. They just keep me confused and worried. So, each time one of those kind comes into my mind I try to catch myself thinking it and say, "No, that's not true," and bring up a different thought, an image of something calm to counteract it. It's helping, but I have to remember to do it. It's amazing how one fear will go and another pop right up to fill the space. I think I create them! I never knew how many fears I've been carrying around all these years.

I've stopped looking at news on TV or reading the paper especially before I go to bed. I don't want to fill myself up with awful stories. I have the habit of paying more attention to bad news than good. I never realized how much of that I took in every day. I've been making a practice this week: every time I think of turning on the TV, I put on some beautiful music instead. I think you love peaceful music best, Baby, but I also love anything that makes me get up and dance.

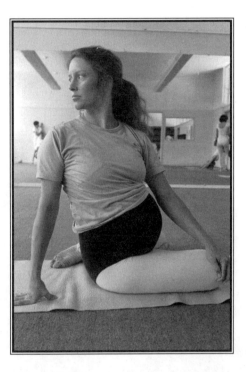

I've been taking a four week movement and dance class. I wonder if I'll make it to the last class on Saturday, I'm feeling so big. But it sure feels wonderful to move my body and stretch a lot. And you always get quiet when I'm dancing, don't you Baby. Are you sleeping, or just wondering what I'm up to and waiting to see what I'll do next?

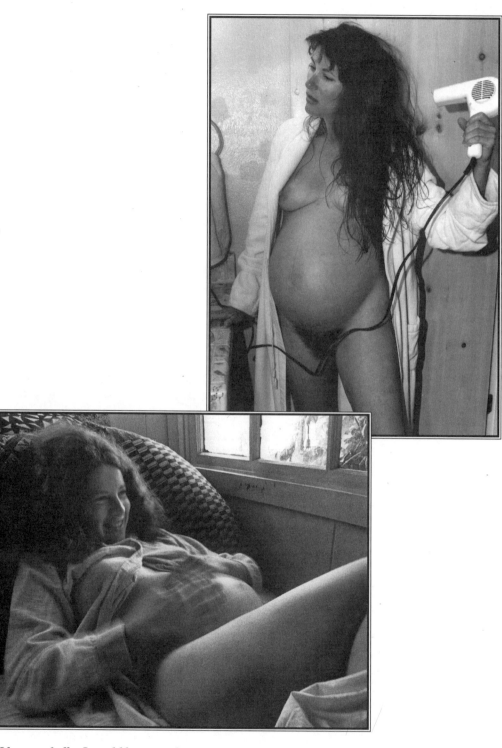

I love my belly. I would love to rub my cheek along it if I could. I'm yummy. Hi, baby. How are you today?

Roxanne says I'm due in five weeks, give or take. She says you can come as soon as next week or wait until two or three weeks after my due date, and we can still have a home birth. But don't come yet, Baby. I'm not ready!

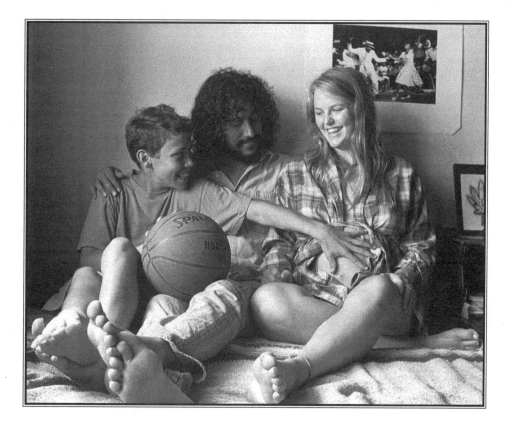

It's funny how everyone talks about her baby being "two days late" or "nine days late," as if the due date is written in stone. I guess it's pretty much like that for cats and some other animals. But are people all the same? Can't some babies take longer?

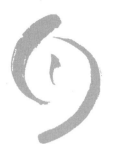

I might as well get all my complaints out at once.

I can't get my belly behind the table when I eat. I have to turn sideways in my chair. I spill everything, like a little kid, down my shirt. I've been having heartburn. I thought that was just something fat men with huge bellies get after eating too much fried food. But I get it almost every time I eat. It feels like heat or fire up high, just under my ribs. Drinking fizzy water helps—makes me burp—and eating only a tiny bit at a time. But I have to sit up straight after each time I eat, or it really hurts.

My bottom ribs have been aching for days, like they're bruised. I called Roxanne today about it. She says it's because I am a bit short-waisted and you are way up under my ribs now, you're getting so big.

You're stretching me out all over, Baby. I'm sorry to complain, but it's getting hard to enjoy being pregnant. It's weird to think I'll never be the same person and my body will never be the same.

I've always had an easy time falling asleep and staying asleep. But now, I can't find any position that's comfortable. I go through this elaborate preparation with pillows, lying on my side and putting one under my belly and another between my knees. Then I'm too hot. I'm hot all the time these days. It's a standing joke between Jay and me. He ends up getting cold and waking up because I kick the blanket off in my sleep. It's actually chilly some nights.

I've been waking up two or three times a night to pee. Sometimes after I pee, when I stand up, I feel like someone has a hand up inside me and is pushing down. It's a sore feeling, like a bruise.

I have spurts of energy, when I feel like I can do everything. Other times, I'm exhausted. My body wants to take a nap every day. But I'm lucky if I can get a few extra breaks at work and go lie down on the couch in the ladies' room.

I'm so insecure these days. I don't believe Jay anymore when he tells me he loves my body. Whenever he mentions a woman at work or lets me know he thinks someone on the TV is attractive, I feel myself getting angry. I've never felt jealousy before. I find myself imagining Jay falling for some slender woman at work who has no kids. Somebody who can wear a string bikini. He better not look at another woman, especially when I'm taking care of our baby. It wouldn't be at all like Jay. Our relationship is built on trust and we've agreed to tell each other if we ever found ourselves thinking about being with someone else. But I hear of so many women whose men had affairs either during the pregnancy or during the first year after the birth!

It's strange how close you can be to someone, yet never know them entirely. Sometimes, when I'm lying in bed, awake, in the middle of the night I wonder, How can you be lying right next to me, and yet we have no idea how each of us is feeling?

Today I'm lumpy and lopsided. The whole center of my body is your territory, Baby. I feel elbows or knees everywhere. I'm getting tired of being pregnant. I've always been physical. Now I get tired when I go on a walk, and get side stitches, and I don't feel safe riding my bike anymore. My bal-

ance is way off. My ankles and wrists swell a bit by the end of the day and my back hurts if I stand around too much.

Stop complaining. This won't last forever. A lot of it is pregnancy hormones. You can tolerate a little discomfort, anxiety and paranoia. It's for a good cause!

You can come now, Baby. Well, not today, but maybe in a week.

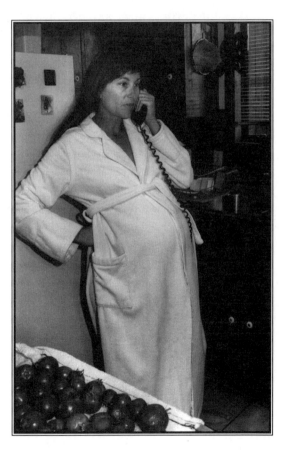

This morning I played hooky from work and went shopping for all the different things Roxanne has asked us to have on hand for the birth. She gave me a list, including lots of those plastic covered pads, to put under me to absorb the fluid. On the list it suggests putting a plastic cover for the mattress under the sheets, when the due date is getting near, in case the membranes rupture. I'll do that when Jay gets home. I want us to get ready together.

I've been trying to find baby clothes and receiving blankets that are all cotton. Everyone says you need at least a dozen receiving blankets, because babies spit up and wet everything. It's not easy to find 100% cotton, but I found some in one of the secondhand stores.

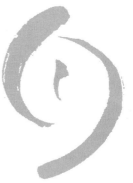

We have to wash a half dozen of them, wrap them in paper bags and tape them shut, then heat them in the oven to sterilize them. It's exciting. I'm glad there are things we have to do to get ready. It's so much more real than just expecting to go to a hospital and have everything taken care of.

This afternoon I washed all the windows in our apartment, inside and out. It wasn't easy. I had to lean way out and my belly kept getting in the way. Jay would have been angry if he saw me. But I just had to do it. I'm having a cleaning frenzy.

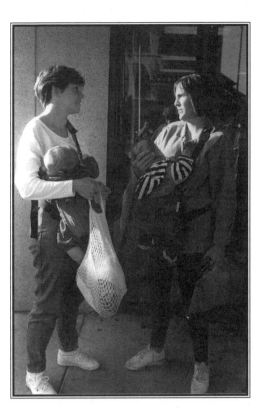

My friends at work are giving me a baby shower this weekend and asked for a list of what we still need. It's fun getting things ready. It gets me thinking about what it will be like when you and *I can go out together, Baby.

Jay's mom and dad are giving us a year of diaper service, so we won't have to use many plastic and paper diapers. They deliver them clean and pick them up dirty! Some things about modern life are great.

Two things I want for sure. I just saw them advertised in a magazine called *Mothering* that I picked up at the natural food store: one is a lamb-skin that is treated so it can be washed, for you to lie on, Baby; the other is a sling to carry you in. There's an article on how in other cultures mothers—or older siblings—have always worn babies close to their body for many months and how babies get a special comfort—and stimulation—from being on someone's body instead of in a baby carrier you push or hold away from your body. I always feel good when I see a guy carrying a baby in a pouch on his chest or in a back pack. I loved reading all the letters to the editor from around the country. I'm feeling like a part of a mini-culture.

Now, the house is clean and we've got everything ready for the birth. You can come now, Baby, even if I'm not quite ready. I've got cold feet!

Roxanne showed me the molded plastic birth stool she brings to all births, because a lot of women find it easier than squatting. She suggested I spend some time alone just feeling out where I might like to give birth in the apartment. It doesn't have to be the bed.

YOUR CHILDREN ARE NOT YOUR CHILDREN. *They are the sons and daughters of Life's longing for itself. They come through you but not from you, and though they are with you, yet they belong not to you. You may give them your love but not your thoughts. For they have their own thoughts. You may house their bodies but not their souls. For their souls dwell in the house of tomorrow, which you cannot visit, not even in your dreams.*

I love that Kahlil Gibran state-ment. I hope I'll be able to remember all that, Baby, when you get me tired and frustrated and I'm feeling angry and not wanting to be a mother. Martie sent me a copy of Gibran's book, *The Prophet*. We had a long talk on the phone last night. We both cried that she can't be here for your birth. But she's planning to come and help over one of the holidays when Jay will be working a lot.

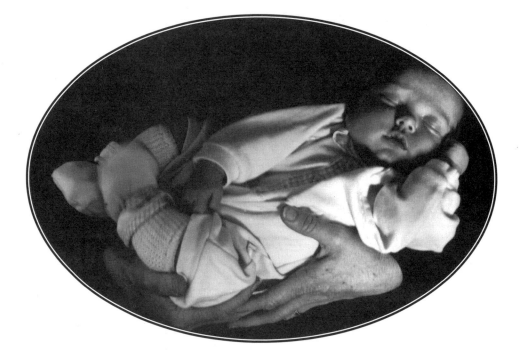

What a great shower! So many pretty things for you, Baby. People were surprised that I don't know what sex you are, since I could know if I let them do the test. But Jay and I are still looking forward to the surprise. We got booties—even a pair of hand-made, beaded, leather, native moc-casins. They're so soft, and so tiny. And we got little sweaters and a bunting for winter. Lots of colors—lavender, green, turquoise, peach, and pale yellow.

Someone gave me a beautiful mobile to hang over the bed for you to watch—patterns of black and white, because new babies are supposed to love that, and they're all hung flat, so you will be able to see them when you're lying on your back, Baby. Several of the women went in together and got me a lambskin and several others the baby carrier I asked for that I saw in the magazine. I'm so lucky, and I feel so grateful.

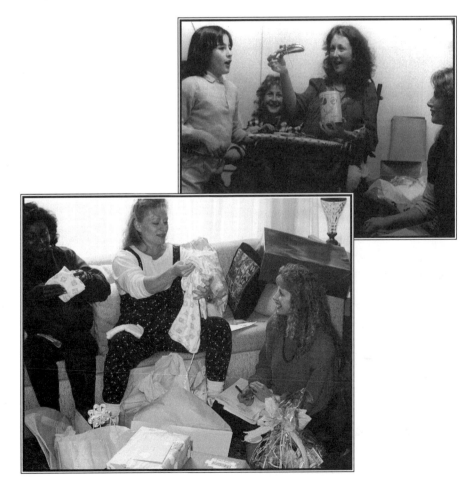

We're having a big summer storm tonight. I love all the lightening and thunder. I remember as a kid in New Jersey, when it would get so hot and humid some nights we couldn't sleep upstairs. So we'd all sleep out on the screened porch. And when a storm came, it was so exciting—and so scary too, the thunder—and then the air would cool down and smell so good afterward.

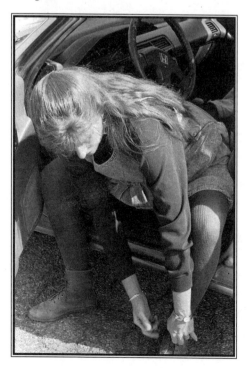

I've been noticing how Jay's and my moods shift when a storm is coming. Especially, if it's been really hot or humid. We get irritable and often have an argument just before the storm begins.

We had an argument because Jay told me his boss wants him to go to a meeting next week that will mean he has to be away for three days. He can drive, but if I go into labor, he'll be three hours away. I told him he couldn't do it. I need him here. I couldn't believe he didn't tell his boss, "No," right off. Jay looked at me like I was crazy when I told him that. He's so used to me feeling independent. "You can reach me by phone." he said. "I'd drive right back." I wish he could know what it's like to feel so insecure right now. He's my lifeline. Sometimes I wish I lived with a whole group of women.

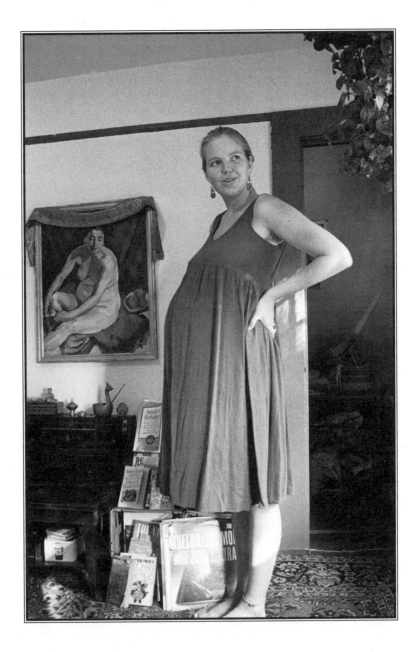

Well, I'm finally waddling like a duck. I read that it's because my pelvic joints are loosening and that it helps make the birth easier. That's great, but I still don't like looking like a duck. My body is not my own.

I have to move my belly to one side and spread my legs to get to my feet to tie my shoes. This is no joke. You're taking over, Baby! But I love you. I can't wait till you're here.

Guess what! My friend Susan came by and told me she wants to do a special women's ceremony for me, with the women I'm closest to, who live nearby, to prepare me for my journey through labor. That's what she called it, your journey. I like that.

I've never heard of a Blessingway. She says it's something a number of Native American tribes traditionally have done whenever someone was about to go on a long journey—including labor. It sounds wonderful. It's going to be a week from Saturday. She asked me to make the list of people to invite. I'm going to include the three women in my birth class. I feel close to them. I also want my sister Melinda to be there if she can drive out. We're very different, but I feel very close to her these days.

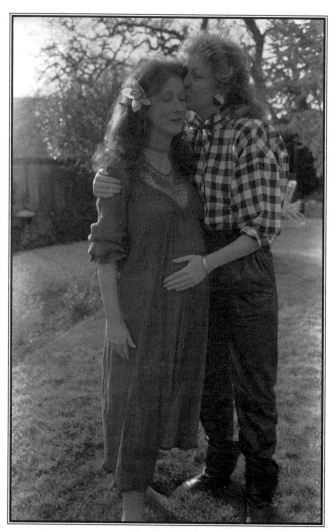

Is my life as an individual coming to an end? I don't even know myself enough yet. Will I be able to take care of you, Baby, the way you deserve? Can I handle all the responsibility? You're going to have to help me.

Yesterday I felt so sure of myself. Today, all that's gone.

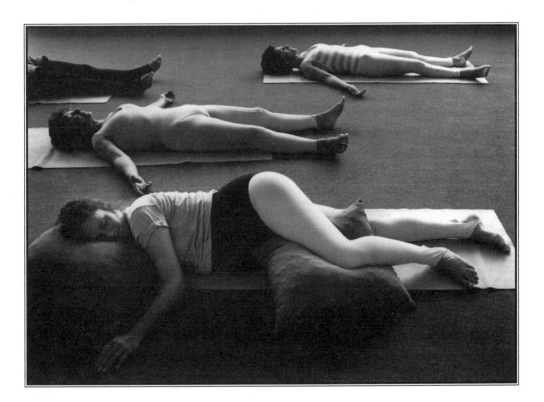

Relax.

I'm pretty sure I want my mom to be with me for this birth. Jay feels good about it too. He understands she and I have something special. She's been great about not asking or inviting herself. I know I'm waiting till the last minute, but... I also wish one of my girlfriends could be there. Susan wants to and she's going to try to arrange her schedule so she can take time off work without notice.

Jay's mom is hinting that she'd love to see her grandchild born. But there's no way. I couldn't let go in labor if she's here. I love her, but she makes me nervous. I've asked Jay to tell her we think we'll need a lot of quiet and privacy after the baby's born and that we'd love to have them come, but they'll need to stay in a motel. He didn't want to be the one to tell them, but I insisted.

It's amazing how many people have never seen a birth and wish they could be there to see what a birth is like, especially without drugs. Even a couple of the guys in Jay's office have hinted they wish they could see it. I wish they could. I think everyone should. But not mine. I'm nervous enough as is. I don't know how I'll be in labor. I need privacy and support. We're thinking about asking Susan or Roxanne's assistant to take pictures. I don't want Jay to. I just want him to be with me.

The sun's just gone down. It was such a beautiful warm day, I didn't want it to end. The days are getting so much shorter. It's too early for summer to end! I don't like darkness right now.

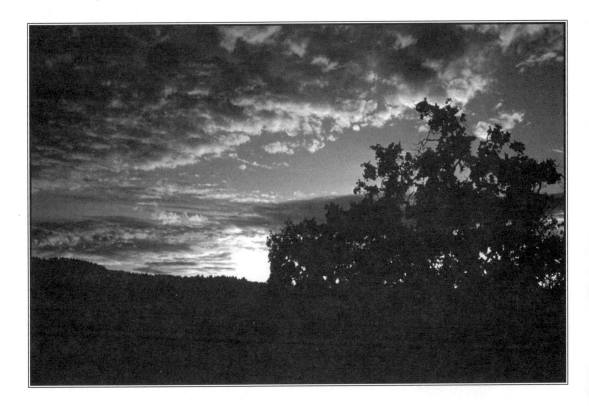

I'm not ready. How could I possibly have thought I could be a good enough mother now? How could I have imagined I could have a home birth?

I've been feeling bad all day, and I couldn't tell why. I closed my eyes and let myself just feel. Suddenly a picture popped into my mind. I'm taking up too much space! I'm out of control. I need this blessing ceremony.

There's so much suffering in the this world. So much pain, especially for so many kids. I'm afraid I'll add to it. I'm afraid I'm just not up to being your mom, Baby. Jay says he sometimes feels that way too. I wish he'd talk about it more. Sometimes I feel so alone. Will you forgive me when I make mistakes and am awful to you, Baby?

I told myself I would never complain about being too big this pregnancy. That's great, in theory. I've gained 41 pounds, and its not just in my belly and breasts! My belly is so round and tight it looks like a gigantic basketball. And the veins on my breasts look like a road map. A woman at work says she got lots of stretch marks in pregnancy, and a dark line from her pubic hair up to her naval. I guess I'm lucky about the stretch marks. I rub cocoa butter on my thighs and breasts and belly every morning and Jay says I smell like a giant chocolate bar. I wonder if that's why I have just a couple of stretch marks on my thighs and the side of my belly. They're red, but Susan said they'll turn white after a while and won't show much. It's sort of a badge, of motherhood, I guess.

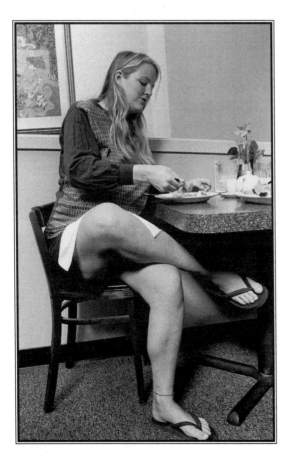

It's getting harder and harder to get a meal down. There just isn't enough room in my stomach. Roxanne showed me a picture of what my insides look like now that you're taking up so much room, Baby. No wonder there's no room for food!

How much longer will I have to wait?

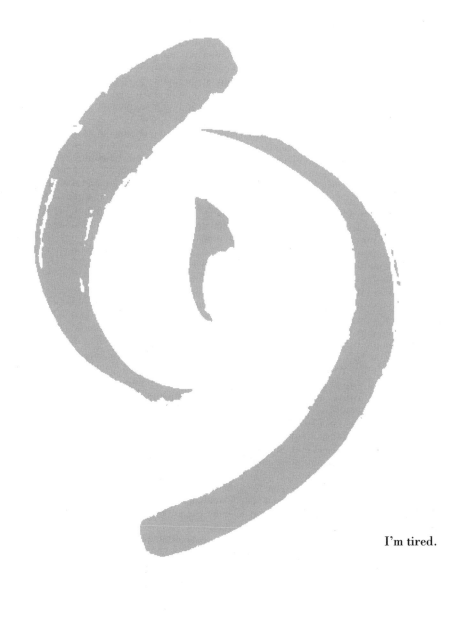

I'm tired.

This morning was my Blessingway. Susan and I decided it should be at dawn and at the park across town because it has a beautiful little grove of redwoods. The weather was perfect. We all sat inside the grove—someone said it's actually a mother tree and all her offspring—in a circle. Everyone was dressed beautifully. Susan brought a Taos drum to beat. It represents the heartbeat of the earth.

Two of my friends painted my belly with symbols that represent the different centers of energy in my body. My sister wore her business clothes and teased me about all my weird friends. I think Jay was a little envious that he wasn't invited, but he was too nice to say so. Some things are just women things.

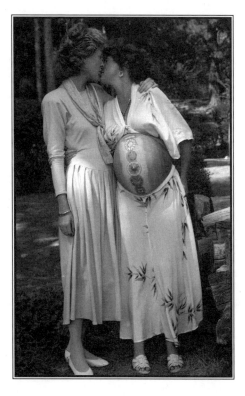

To start, Susan lit a candle and one of the other women prayed to the spirits of my female ancestors and to the spirits who are watching over you and me, Baby. She asked them all to come into the circle and give us direction and clarity. The drumbeat felt good in my body, like a slow, deep pulse. Four of the women washed my feet in a bowl of warm water filled with flower blossoms and herbs. Susan talked about the journey I am on, the long walk I must make on my own to birth you, Baby. Two of the women from class brushed my hair and pinned it up. I almost always wear it down, so she said putting it up symbolized the change in my life that is to come with your arrival, Baby.

or clean house for us in the first two weeks. That's so Jay and I can put all our attention on the three of us just getting to know each other.

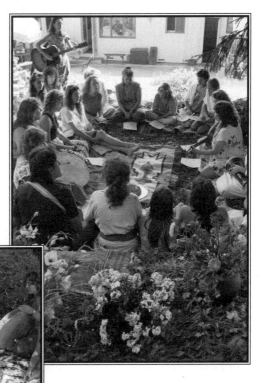

Each of the women in turn gave me her blessing, wished me strength, or good humor, or flexibility, or courage, or trust. I really felt their wishes enter me. They gave me a gift certificate for four massages—one for every week after the birth. And one of the women said she would organize all my friends and people I work with to bring Jay and me food or run errands

I feel so honored. And different. I'll never forget it—the feeling of being in that circle of women. Tonight I'm going to finish the tape I've been making of the music I love most, to listen to in labor. Nothing too loud or fast, just music to keep me calm and keep me going.

At our last birth class we watched a movie that was nothing but a series of deliveries, just the few seconds before the actual birth and through the delivery. Every one of the mothers were squatting. It was filmed in a South American hospital where they discovered how much better the births went if the mother walked around in labor and squatted for birth. Our teacher said that x-ray studies of the pelvis proved that when a woman squats her pelvis actually expands. People say it's bone, so it's rigid, but it's not—it's jointed. I couldn't believe these births! The babies just slipped right out onto the bed. No one's hands were even in the picture! I can't get the images out of my mind. You really *can* come out of my body. Amazing!

One of the women in class was induced for her first birth because her doctor thought her water might have broken. Our birth teacher said it was probably what they call "a high leak," and that her body would most likely have sealed it closed. But her doctor didn't wait to find out. Because there was amniotic fluid,

after 24 hours when her labor hadn't started on its own, he insisted on inducing her with artificial hormones. Our teacher said that was still the rule in most hospitals, even though studies had proven that waiting for the labor to begin on its own doesn't increase the risk to the baby.

Anyway, this woman, Elena, ended up with everything she and her husband hadn't wanted. Once they started, it was one thing after another. She wanted her coach to be her advocate, but the coach didn't feel she could stand up to the nurses and her doctor. Later on Elena said she did a lot of reading and going over her medical records with other people and it was pretty clear she was sure she could have had a perfectly normal birth if they hadn't started interfering.

She told us she took an epidural because they offered it when she was right in the middle of a hard contraction and feeling hopeless. Then she wasn't able to feel enough to push well. Plus, the baby got stuck and they had to pull him out with a vacuum machine. They took him away to the nursery for observation but they ended up doing all sorts of things to him just because he was in the nursery. She said that's why she came to this class and didn't go to the free classes at the hospital. I felt angry and sad for her. I hope she has a good birth this time.

The last part of class was the best. One of the couples was missing, because they'd had their baby last Tuesday. They surprised us by coming the last half hour. They brought the baby. The teacher asked if we could stay late so we could hear about their birth. Marcia told us all about her labor. It was in the hospital and they had wanted to give her drugs to speed up labor. She refused and her husband told the nurse they needed some time alone. When they were alone they turned off the lights and her husband sucked on her breasts to make contractions get stronger. She said they did. It was something she read about in a book, that nipple stimulation of any kind brings on the same hormone that produces labor contractions. At first she felt a bit embarrassed, but she really wanted a natural birth, and it worked. Good for her!

She said labor was the hardest work she'd every done, and she could not have gotten through without her husband. At one point she said, "I can't do this!" And he put his hands around her face, looked her straight in the eyes and said very calmly, "You *know* you can." He told us that he was really a bit afraid himself, only he was determined not to let her see it. She said it was just the thing she needed to go on. She was at 9 centimeters. Our teacher said transition can be the hardest time, because contractions sometimes come back-to-back and a woman can feel confused and overwhelmed and then get frightened. Marcia only pushed for forty-five minutes, because she remembered what she learned in class and had David hold her under her armpits so she could squat. She didn't tear at all, and even her doctor was surprised! I'm so glad I'm around people who I can talk to about these things and get ideas from. Their baby is gorgeous! He has the most beautiful, long fingers and big dark eyes. He was so alert. And Marcia and David are so in love with him. It's been great watching David change from being super analytical to a real softie.

I'm sorry birth classes are over. I've really liked having a special time each week I could look forward to getting together with people who are as interested as we are in talking about birth and babies. We're going to have a reunion before Thanksgiving, after we've all had our babies.

Finally, I feel this is real.

Mom is so excited. I asked her to be at the birth. She's going to drive out to be here a week before the due date. If I go into labor before that, she says she'll get on the first plane. I told her our place is so small, I need her to stay somewhere else. She understood. She doesn't have money for a motel, so Susan said she could stay at their house. I'm really glad. People are being so helpful. I've had to learn to ask for what I need.

❀

I've been thinking about what it will be like after you're here, Baby. One of the women in class was talking about how hard it was for her after she got home from the hospital with their first baby, because her relatives kept coming to stay with them and friends kept dropping by. She said everyone said they just wanted to see the baby and said they wanted to help, but most of them didn't know how to be helpful. So she ended up entertaining everyone. And she got a breast infection, which her pediatrician said was from doing too much and not nursing often enough.

It's so hard to say no to people who just want to see the baby and con-

gratulate us. But Roxanne, Mom and Susan are both reminding me that in the first weeks I need to be selfish, because my body will need time to rest and recover.

Jay and I have talked about it. We want to keep our place really quiet and have a lot of privacy in the first weeks.

I talked to Roxanne about visitors after the birth and she showed me a sign Kate made up for couples to put on their door. It says,

> *"Thanks for coming by. Sara and the baby are fine. They need all the quiet and rest they can get. Please understand why we're not taking visitors today. But we'd love it if you want to leave a note or some food or flowers. We'll call you when we're ready for visitors."*

Jay and I are going to make a sign and put the same message on our answering machine after the birth.

And we need to be protective of you, Baby, since babies don't like to be handled by just *anyone*, especially people who don't know how to be with a new baby's sensitive energy.

Roxanne says a new mother and baby are wide open and that they need a circle of protection around them. She suggests I consider staying inside for a month, if I can do it, because the special feeling from the birth disappears so easily, when you go out into the world too soon, and are around all the noisy energy that's out there.

Everyone I know seems to be proud of how soon they went out with the baby, how soon they got back into their routine.

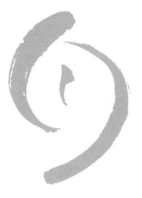

Roxanne suggested I stay in my bathrobe and nightgown or pajamas for as many days as possible, because people—including Jay—won't expect me to be back into my whole routine then, the way they will if I get dressed every morning. She's got six kids, four of them step-kids. She told me what it was like for her after each of her two births, and how, when she went out the first time—to an exercise class, with the baby—it was too soon. She didn't know till she got home and burst into tears. That was when she realized her home was a safe cocoon, and that she needed to be there a little longer. Why don't women talk about things like this?

Baseball season is coming to an end. The leaves are turning colors. I love it. The smell of fall. The sound of the sports announcer on the radio during the game just now brought back so many memories of the end of summer as a kid.

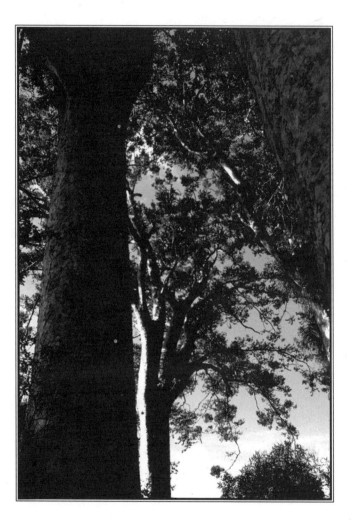

Baby, you've been quieter than usual for a couple of days. Are you tired, too? Or just resting up for the big day?

A few mornings when I've woken up there's been yellowish dried stuff on my nipples. I read about it. It's colostrum for you, Baby! It's very rich and creamy. I read that in some cultures women are superstitious about it and won't let their babies take the colostrum. But it's *good* for babies.

I wonder what breastfeeding will feel like.

I asked Roxanne about lovemaking. Would it hurt you, Baby, now that you're so big inside me? I'm still turned on, but Jay is worried. Roxanne said the amniotic sac you are living in and the fluid around you is a protection from injury. She also said that a lot of women go into labor after having intercourse—if their baby is ready—because there's a hormone called prostaglandin in semen that softens a woman's cervix and can help get labor started.

She gave me copies of three articles to read—one on sex and pregnancy and sex after birth, one on natural labor aids, and one on postpartum care of my body. I didn't know that having an orgasm can bring on labor and that it can be a way to get labor going if a baby is more than a week or two past due date, to avoid getting induced. Babies apparently only have a problem with their mother having intercourse if

it's rough or something she's doing against her desire. A baby is sensitive to what its mother is feeling, even in the womb. It also talks about masturbation as a good way to get labor started, or get early labor to kick into active labor. That sounds weird. I don't know if I could do it, especially if I had to be in the hospital.

The article on natural labor aids suggests a variety of things to pick up a very slow or stuck labor, or induce a very late labor. Most of them I learned in class: taking walks and hot showers, eating whatever you feel like, getting lots of fluids, getting massage, having acupuncture needles in special places or pressing on pressure points with the thumb. I learned some more about handling pain, like how to stimulate the pleasure center of the brain, since that diminishes the sensation of pain: looking at beautiful things, hearing music you love, being touched in ways that feel good. Staying up and moving around as much as possible has been found to make contractions more efficient and shorter. I'm all for that! Roxanne gave me her and Kate's list of books they recommend on postpartum for me and baby care and child development. I'm off to the library to see what they have.

Jay and I got up early and took a long walk as the sun was coming up today. The days are getting shorter. On the way back, we weren't talking, just holding hands, and a name just appeared in my mind. A girl's name. I've wondered what you wanted us to call you, Baby. Jay agreed, that should be your name. What do you think of the name Molly? Of course, we'd better pick out a boy's name, too. I like Michael.

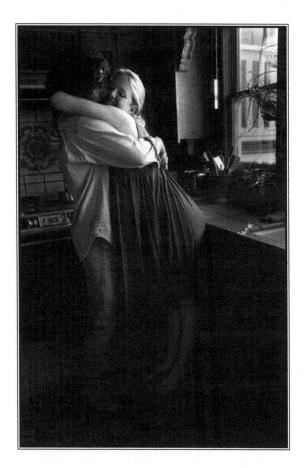

My belly button is stretched flat now. I wonder if it's going to pop out. There's a piece of dark lint that's been in my navel ever since I can remember. Today I was finally able to pull it out!

I've been having a few contractions—they're called Braxton-Hicks and they're not real labor contractions, but they are getting my uterus ready for labor. It's a tightening low down in my belly and going all the way down into my inner thighs. It almost feels like a muscle cramping. Roxanne suggested I drink some herb tea, raspberry leaf, to strengthen my uterus. I just read that the uterus is the strongest muscle in the body! It's going to be doing lots of work in labor.

I have no idea what real labor contractions will feel like. Is the pain like someone punching you or like a stabbing pain? Some women say it's like period cramps, but I've never had cramps with my period, just aching in my lower back. It's hard to be too scared of something I have no idea of.

The idea of tearing still scares me. One of the women in class who refused an episiotomy for her first birth did tear, but she says it was no big deal and didn't hurt at the time, there was so much else going on, and it healed quickly. Today Roxanne asked me about my last-minute fears and I told her it was tearing. She said if I do, it will happen along the line of least resistance, *after* the perineum has stretched very thin. So it's more like a cut at the corner of your mouth, and heals more quickly than a scissor cut. That's been proven. Also, there are herbs I can put in a shallow bath to help the healing. That made me feel a bit better.

Roxanne says the women she's seen tear are those whose labor is so fast at the end that they can't focus on letting the baby just slip out slowly, in between contractions, the way she likes to have them do to prevent a tear. When she worked in the hospital she saw a lot of third and fourth degree episiotomies—that's where the cut extends through the rectum. Ouch! The worst she has seen as a midwife is a second degree.

Martie called. A friend of hers found an obstetrician who really likes natural childbirth, and she had an 11 pound first baby with him without tearing.

I've noticed that women say, "Doctor so-and-so delivered my baby." Why not, "*I* delivered my baby"?

When I think about tearing, I'll imagine instead my perineum opening like a flower—like the water lily I saw. I'll picture my body stretching all around your head, Baby, and you just *slipping* out.

The sky is bleak and the clouds are low this morning. It's going to rain. I'm all alone.

Jay's gone to work. I'm playing hooky. I'm going to make myself a wonderful breakfast and fix up a tray and eat it in bed—very slowly. I deserve a treat.

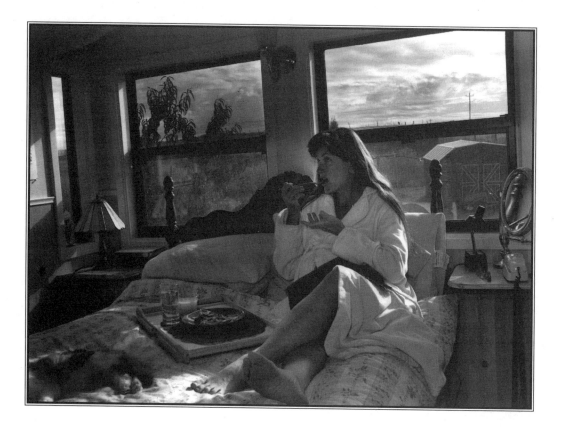

Susan just told me a high school friend of hers wrote her and told her she had a water birth. She saw a film about it in pregnancy, and actually found a hospital that had just gotten a big tub for women to use in labor.

The baby was born in water. Amazing. I wish I'd heard about having a water birth earlier. But I'm happy with my plans.

Sometimes, *having* to wait, knowing this is something that will happen in its own time, is a *good* feeling. Knowing that it's not up to me. You'll come when you're ready.

It's getting so close. Sometimes it feels like this pregnancy is taking forever. Other times it feels like it's whizzing by.

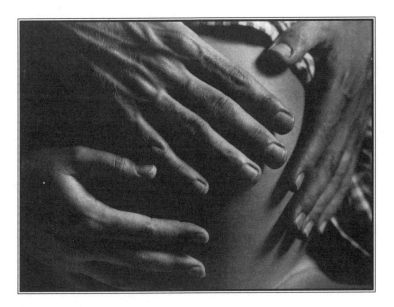

I'm going to miss you, belly. I hope that in labor I'll be able to get my mind out of the way and just let my body do its work. I'm sure it knows what to do better than my mind.

I woke up early this morning, before dawn. There's a strong wind. Fall is here. I get a bit melancholy each year at this time. I hate to see this summer end, but I do love the change of seasons. I lay and listened to the wind and watched the stars and moon fade—it's almost full again—as the sky grew light. How much longer will I have to wait? What will it be like?

What will you be like, Baby?

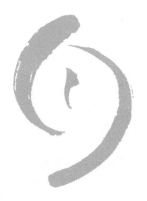

Last night I woke up in the middle of the night and felt a bit nauseous. I did not want to be awake alone, so I woke up Jay. We drank chamomile tea and played music and talked. He massaged my back where it's sore. It was a very special time together. But this morning he woke feeling sick. I think it's a flu. What if I get a flu just before I go into labor? Does it ever happen?

You know what your heartbeat sounds like, Baby? Like a humming bird beating your wings. Almost twice as fast as mine.

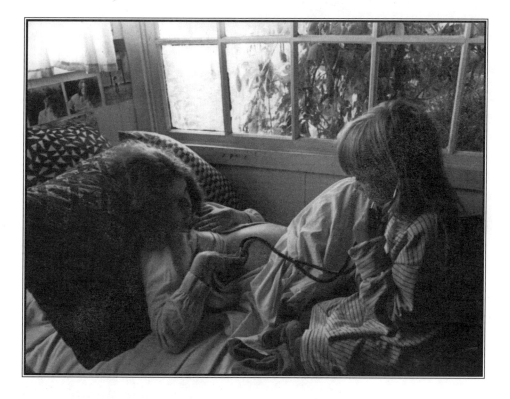

Hooray! My cervix is most of the way thinned—effaced. It won't be long now.

Sometimes it seems as if I've been pregnant all my life. I can't remember not being pregnant.

I think I'm in labor!

They feel like waves coming over me. Feels so good when it ends, and I can catch my breath.

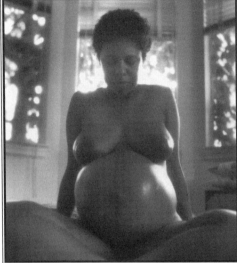

Long hot shower. The warm water feels so good on my back. I could stay here forever.

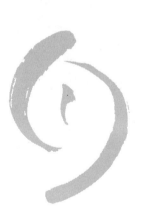

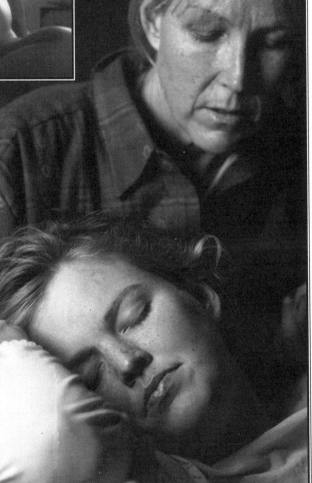

I'm so glad Susan and Jay and my mom are here.

Jay, don't leave the room. I need you every minute.

I'm thirsty.

What do they mean, "Relax"!

Susan and my mom massaging my feet and my hands and my thighs.

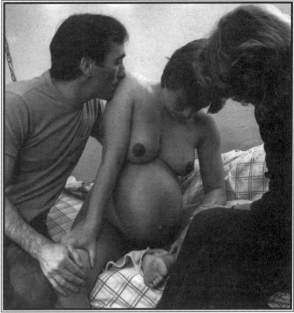

Ooooh. That helps.

Do I *have* to drink some more?

It's taking too long. Now I know why some women ask for drugs!

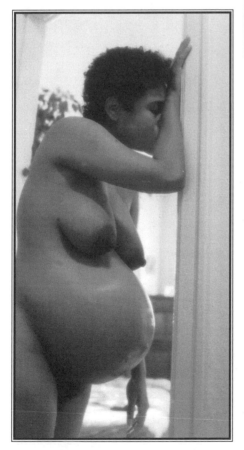

Feel so sorry for myself. This is too much. And it's taking too long!

Have to stay on my feet. Even sitting hurts. Lying down is excruciating!

Don't talk to me in the middle of a contraction!

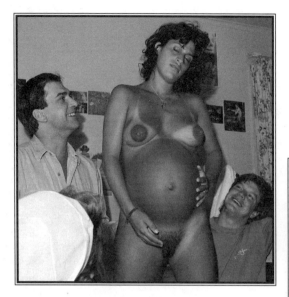

I'm too tired to stand up. Rocking back and forth on my hands and knees feels good.

Come on, Baby. Please! Oh, please.

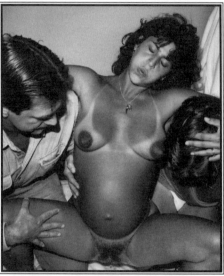

I'm hot. Now I'm cold.

Oh, God. Oh, God.

Don't touch me!

Crying. Something let go inside me just now.

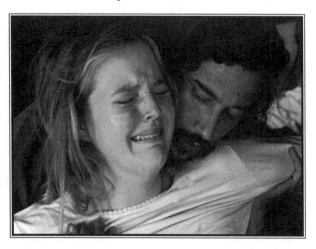

Oh, shit. Oh, shit. Oh, God.

How much longer?

I'm so tired.

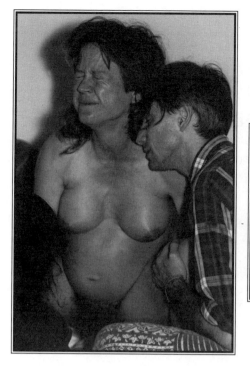

Ooooh. The waters broke. What a relief! The contractions keep coming back-to-back. There's no rest.

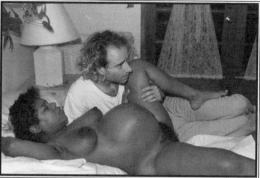

Don't make me move!

I have to *push!*

I can't. Do something.

Will I split open? Ooooh.

I feel like something's coming out. I have to shit.

Something hot and wet on my perineum. Ooooh. It helps the burning.

Ooooh. Hurts.

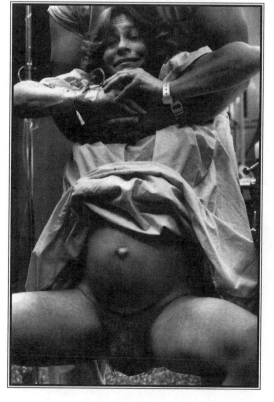

Oh, Baby. Baby. Baby. Pleeeease.

You're here! It's you. You're really here!

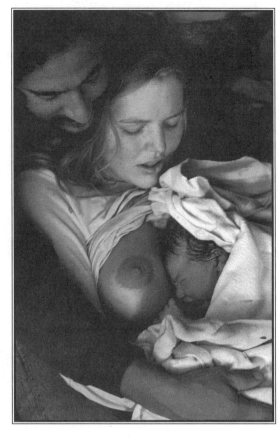

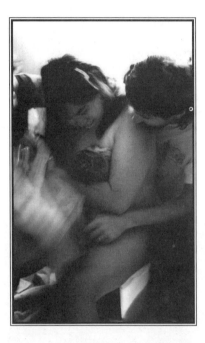

Hello, Baby. I love you.

What? I have to push again? For my placenta? Will you hold her so I can concentrate on pushing?

It's out. No more pushing!

That's where you lived. What a big placenta.

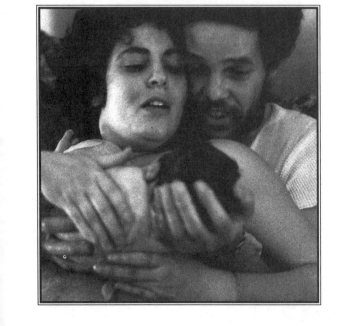

So *that's* your umbilical cord. It's so slippery and tough.

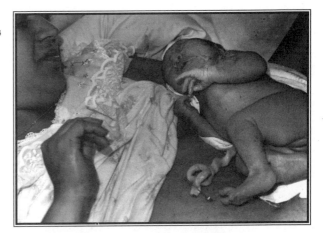

Are you tired after all your work?

Let's cover you with a nice, warm blanket, so you don't get a chill.

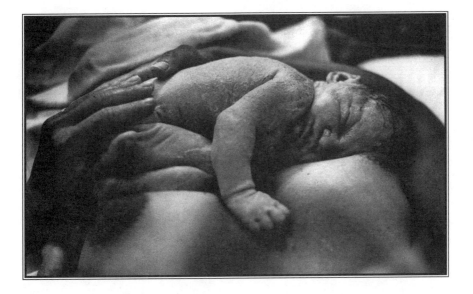

Is that what vernix is? It's so creamy. Feel her skin. It's velvet.

Did I shout as loud as I think I did?

I'm so hungry!

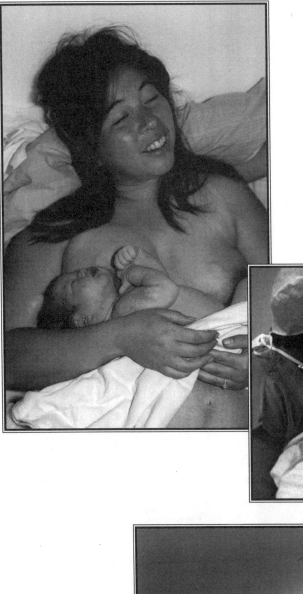

I did it! We *did* it!

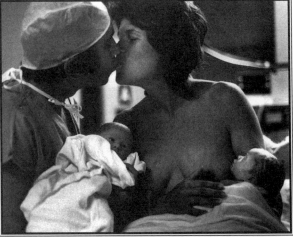

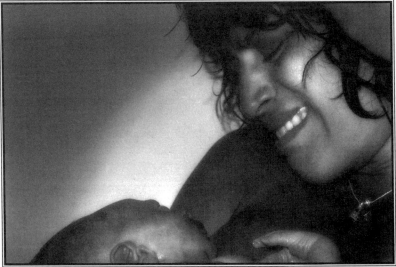

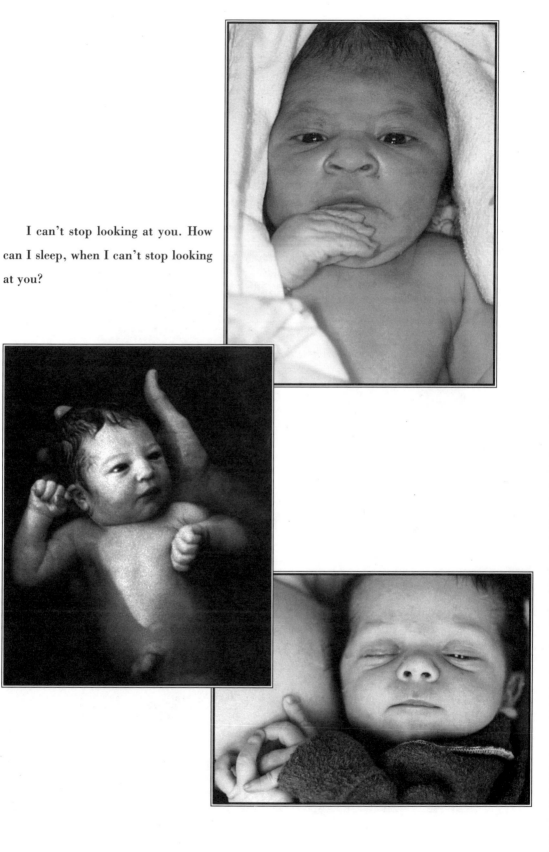

I can't stop looking at you. How can I sleep, when I can't stop looking at you?

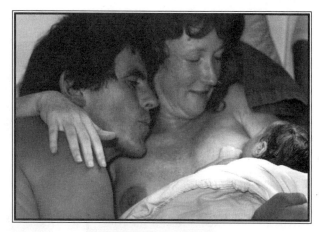

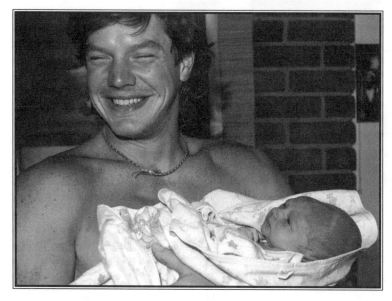

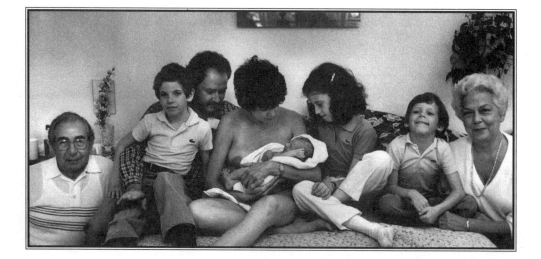

The meconium: so slippery and black.

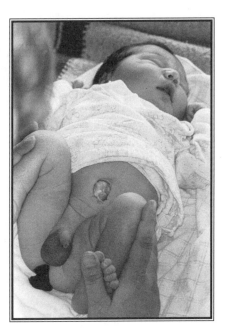

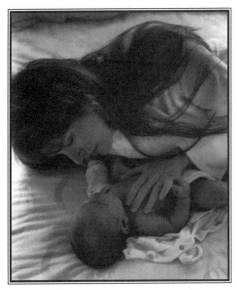

Poor Baby. You've got hiccups.

Your cord: I don't want your diaper to rub against it and make it bleed or hurt you.

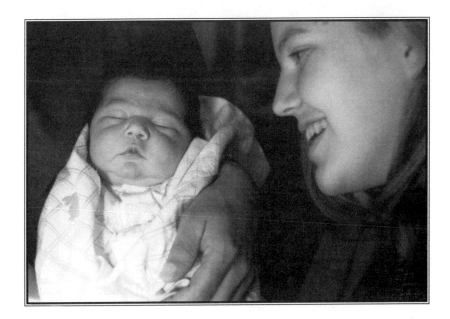

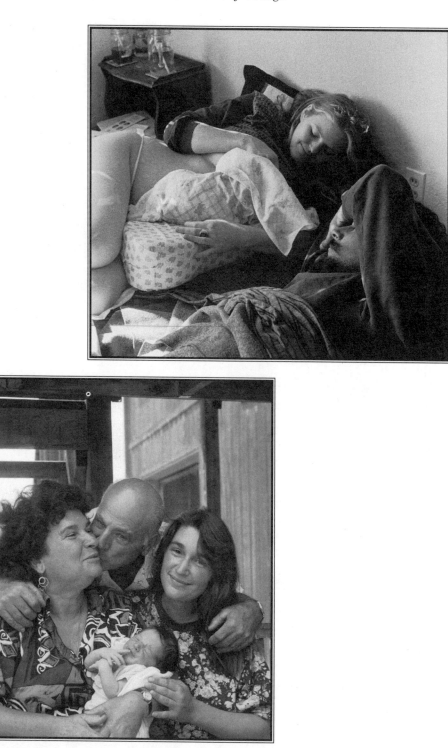

The sun was so warm this afternoon, I got dressed and we all went outside for a family picture. Three generations.

My belly. It's so squishy.

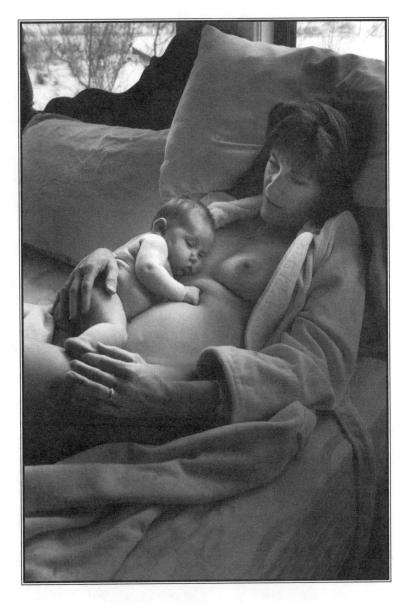

You're so perfect. How could any-

one so perfect come out of my body?

Sometimes, when you are sleeping, you move your hands like pictures I've seen of a Balinese dancer.

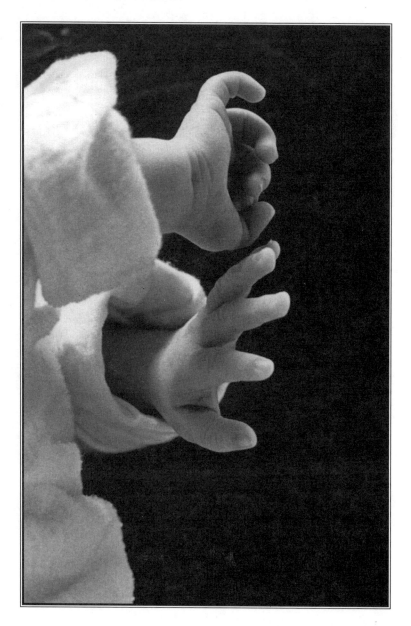

I'm hardly sore at all. Your head felt *so* big when you were coming out. But I only have a few "skid marks." We got a little spray bottle that I fill it with warm water to use instead of wiping.

Your cord stump fell off today when I was changing your diaper. I remember someone saying that in some tribal cultures part of a baby's cord or the cord stump is kept in a little pouch for the baby. It's considered sacred, a protection for that person, that they keep with them forever.

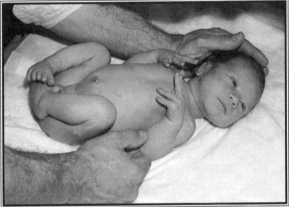

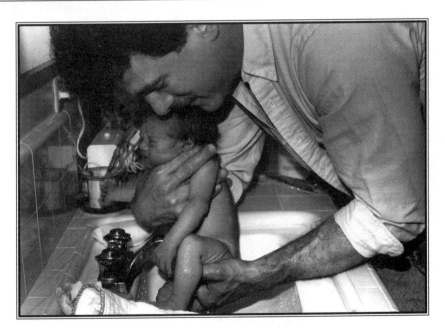

We just gave you your first bath. You screamed, but then you liked it. You're so slippery when you're wet. I was afraid your head would slip under the water. We're so awkward, Baby. Please be patient with us.

You've been nursing and crying all night. *Nothing* we do seems to make you feel better. I'm so tired. What can we do?

It seems like one feed ends and you want to begin again.

I'm so glad everyone's bringing us food. Some people are even bringing whole meals. How do women who are all alone do it? I wish everyone had this much attention.

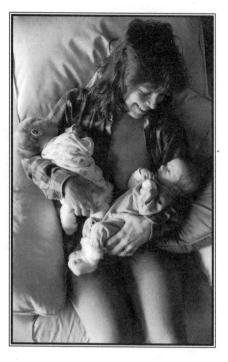

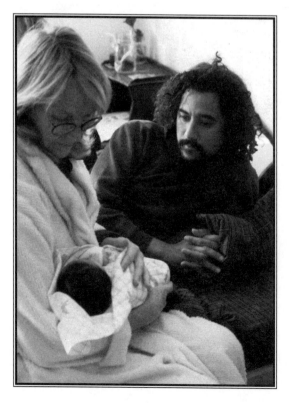

Roxanne stopped by for a post-partum visit. She says we're doing great, that it's just going to take some time for all of us to get adjusted to each other. She reminded me that breastfeeding can take some practice in the first couple weeks, but once it's going well, it will be so easy.

I'm so glad Mom stayed over last night. How can one little baby take up all the attention of three adults?

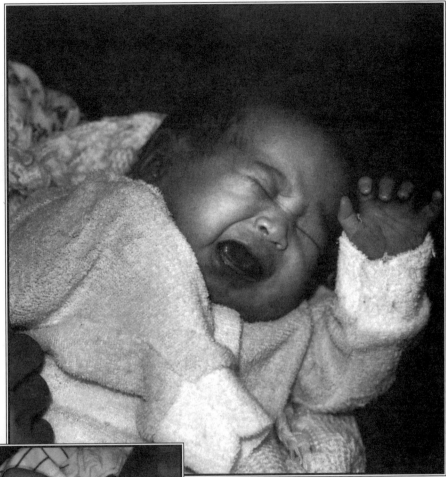

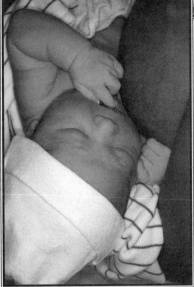

I can't understand your crying. I'm trying to learn what each of your cries means. Do you get as frustrated as I do?

I called the La Leche League today. I wasn't sure I've been positioning you correctly on my breast, because it still hurts sometimes when you latch on, and sometimes you feed forever.

A woman named Marcia is coming over this afternoon to watch an entire feeding and give me suggestions if I need them. I'm so glad.

Marcia reminded me to have your body tucked in really close and to wait until your mouth is wide open before I let you take my breast. That's all it took for it not to hurt!

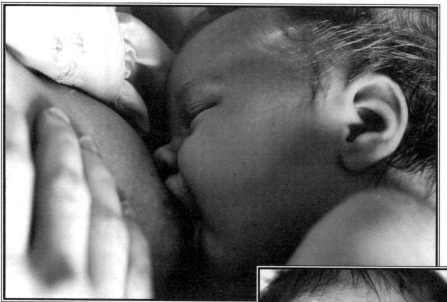

You had a great feeding and fell sound asleep after you came off my breast.

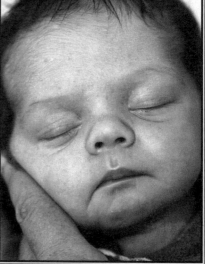

Isn't it amazing that you can nurse and breathe at the same time. I love the sounds you make while you nurse.

You just raised your arm way up over your head, and I discovered a bit of vernix in your armpit left from the birth.

Milk. Dripping everywhere! I'm leaking from both ends.

When my milk dries on my nightgown, it feels like cement.

Kate dropped by. She was in the neighborhood. I miss her and Roxanne. Especially Roxanne. We were so close in pregnancy. Now she has other women to care for, and I envy them.

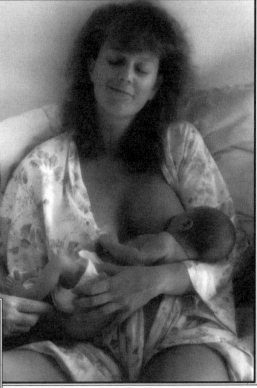

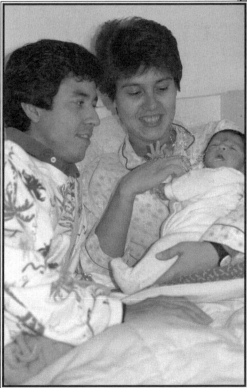

I have *so* much energy! People talk so much about postpartum blues. What about postpartum *bliss*!

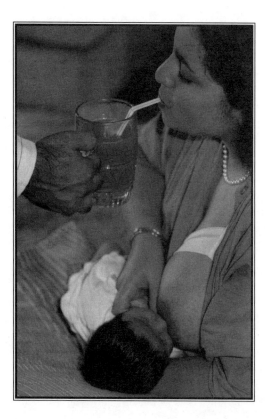

It's good to have mom still here,
and it's good when she goes to Susan's
at night, so we can be alone.

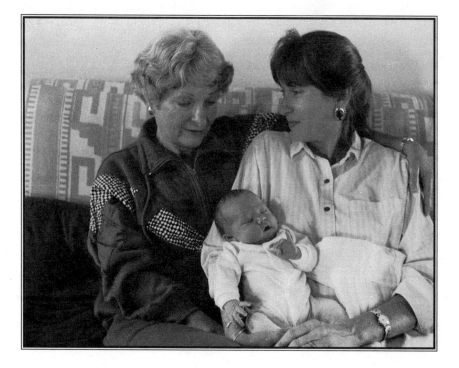

We had to leave the apartment today to see the pediatrician for a full check-up. I wish pediatricians made home visits, like midwives do.

Jay drove us. You looked so tiny strapped into the infant seat we got for the car.

I like Jane's (the pediatrician's) way with a baby. After examining

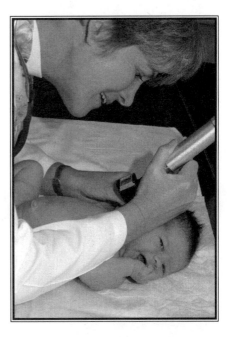

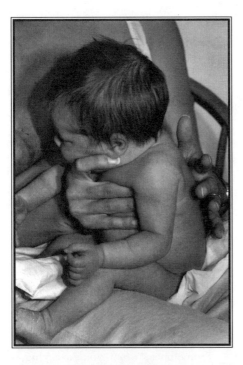

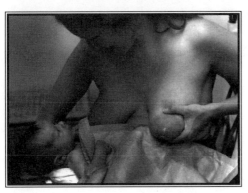

you, she showed me an easy way to bring up air in your tummy after feeding. I sit you up over one of my hands to support your chest, and gently rub your back.

She told me all about the healing properties of breast milk. Besides giving you protective antibodies, breast milk can even be dropped in a baby's eye to heal an infection. She also showed me how to express my milk, so Jay can feed you if I need to be away from you. I don't need a pump; it just takes practice. Right now, I don't want to leave you at all, not for a minute. You're a part of me. I *want* to be with you.

My left nipple is sore. I'm wondering whether you're latching on to enough of my breast when I nurse you in the middle of the night, because I'm not as careful then. I have to pay more attention.

When you cry, my breasts tingle, like there's electricity in them. Sometimes, when I'm not holding you, just thinking about you makes my milk drip!

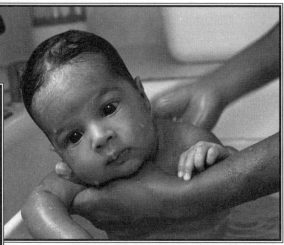

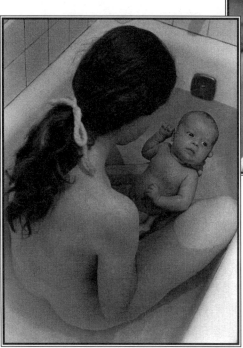

Sometimes, when you're crying, everyone else seems able to get you calm but me! I get jealous. I'm still awkward at this mothering business. Be patient, Baby.

Last night was the first time I could get you to feed easily while I was lying on my side. It was wonderful being able to get you started, and then being able to sleep while you nursed.

Jay was worried about our sleeping with you in our bed. You're in the middle. I know we wouldn't roll over on you, but I called the pediatrician just to check. She agreed with me. And it's so nice, being in bed all together.

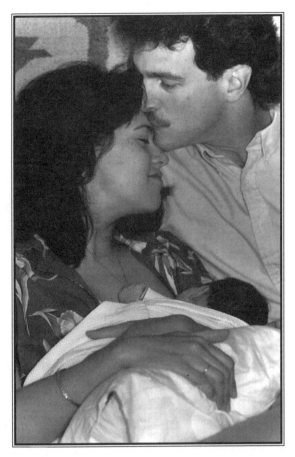

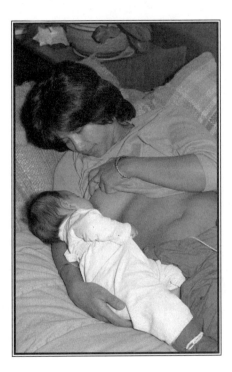

I'm eating for two. I can eat anything I want, because I'm breastfeeding, and I'm losing weight anyway. My belly still feels like jello, though. Time to start exercising. Now that you and I have got the hang of it, breastfeeding sure is easy, and it's free.

Last night I just took you into the living room each time you cried, so Jay could get some sleep. Jay's parents got us a lovely rocking chair with a tall back. I rocked you for a long time, and sang to you all the songs I remember Mom singing to me. I felt connected with every mother on the planet who was rocking her baby to sleep. It felt so safe and far away from everything.

You love your lambskin. You lie on it and ball your fist in the soft fur.

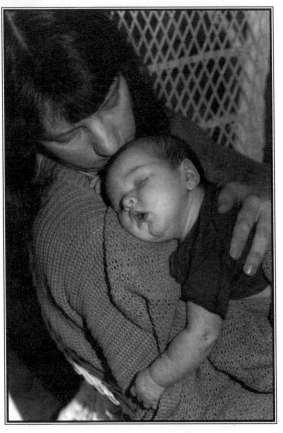

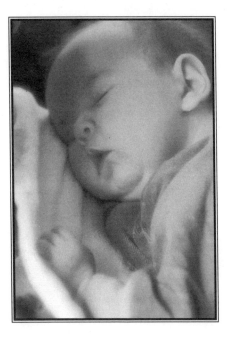

Jay hinted last night that he'd like to make love. I don't have the desire yet. I'm afraid I might be sore inside. Also, having you feed so often and being so much a part of my body still, I am full up with being touched. For now. But I want to give something to Jay He's been so wonderful. Perhaps tonight. We can take it very slowly.

I don't want to leave the apartment today. It's raining and cold outside and so snug in here with you, Molly.

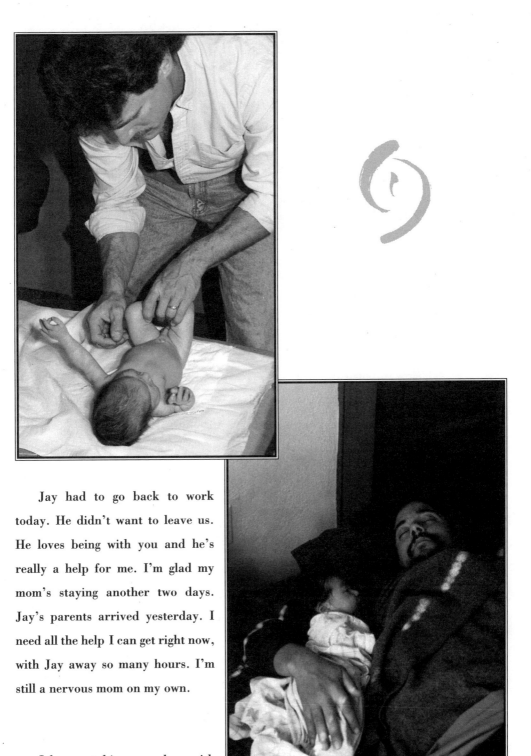

Jay had to go back to work today. He didn't want to leave us. He loves being with you and he's really a help for me. I'm glad my mom's staying another two days. Jay's parents arrived yesterday. I need all the help I can get right now, with Jay away so many hours. I'm still a nervous mom on my own.

I love watching you sleep with your Daddy.

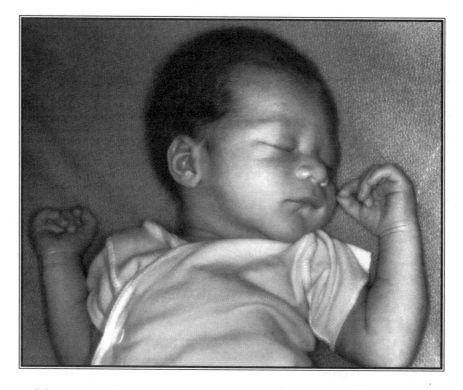

I have so much to learn, I don't know what you're trying to tell me a lot of the time when you cry. Sometimes it really seems like a tummy ache or gas. You draw your legs up. Other times you seem to want to feed, but when I show you my breast and bring your face to it, you turn your head as if you don't want it and cry.

I have discovered that you like to have your arms free sometimes and other times you want to be swaddled in a blanket, with your arms across your chest, and just your head out. Do you feel more secure like that? I'm reading all the baby books I can, but it's nice to be able to call someone from the breastfeeding group when I have questions.

Susan's been wonderful. She knows just how to be with me, and she's wonderful with a baby.

We've begun to let people visit for a short time. But I won't let everyone hold you, just people who feel right. At first it was hard for me to refuse someone saying, "Can I hold her?" Now I say, "Now's not a good time. I'm enjoying holding her." What can they say? Jay and I've talked about it. It's up to us to protect you.

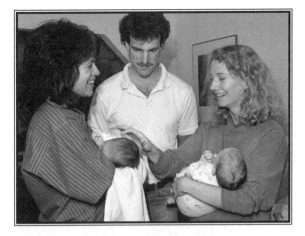

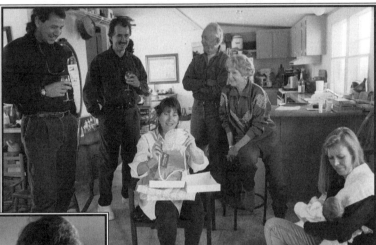

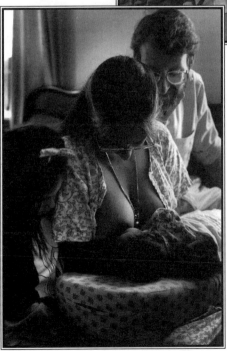

We were given an illustrated book called *Infant Massage*. I can't wait to try it. It's supposed to be especially healing for babies who've had difficult births. I think your birth was easy—if you can call *any* birth easy. But according to this book, any baby loves and benefits from being massaged.

This afternoon I was tense and snapped at Jay after he got home from work. You'd been crying a lot and I was tired, and he was tired from work. So I decided to try taking a shower with you. I ran the water warm enough for you—that's cooler than I like, but you're not ready for hot water. Your skin's too tender.

At first you seemed nervous—your arms flew out and your eyes were big in surprise. But I held you real tight against my breast, with both arms across your body, and gradually I turned so your body was under the water. You began to relax and then started to lick the water off my skin. I cried. It was so wonderful.

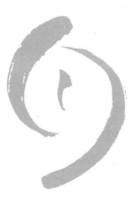

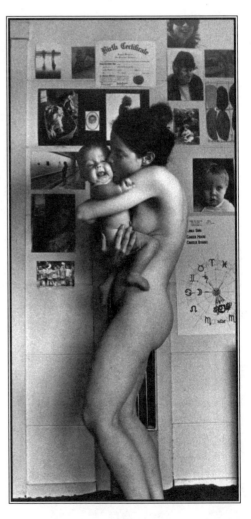

Jay took pictures of me nude today. It's for posterity. What will my breasts look like when you're done nursing on me, Molly?

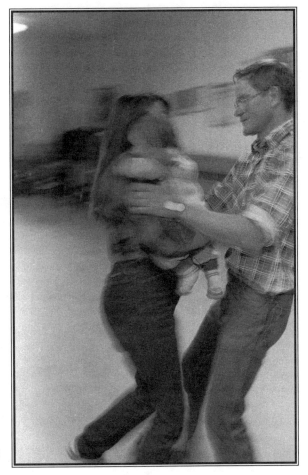

Jay and I decided to take you out into the world today. Your first journey in public. We couldn't think where would be special enough. Then we decided to go to the conservatory of flowers at the park, where I loved to go during pregnancy. On the way to the car, an old lady stopped us to admire our baby.

When I left the apartment—it's been almost 28 days—just stepping outside on the pavement the world looked magical. I'm glad I took this month just to be in our little cave.

I think you loved the smells and especially the moist, warm air in the orchid room, as much as I do. Jay carried you in the sling and looked so proud. I felt like dancing.

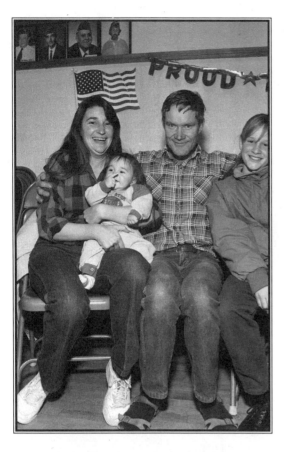

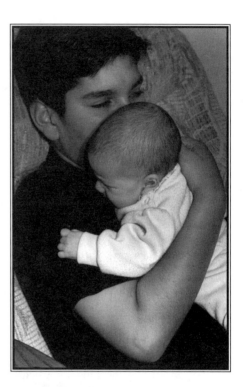

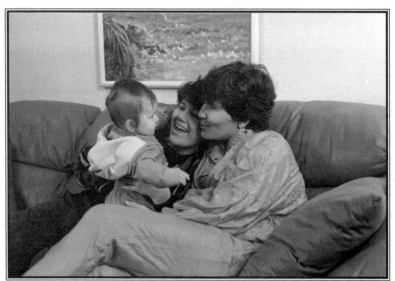

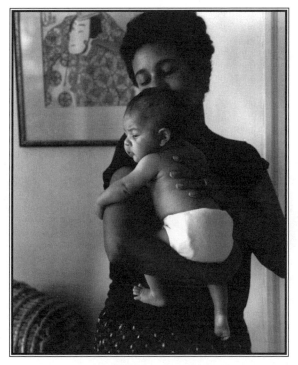

Today we had a family ceremony to plant your placenta—we've been keeping it in the freezer—in the earth beneath a baby evergreen your dad bought to celebrate your coming into our family. We thought of putting it in our yard, but you know how often people move these days. So, we planted it along a trail in the state park, where you can always find it.

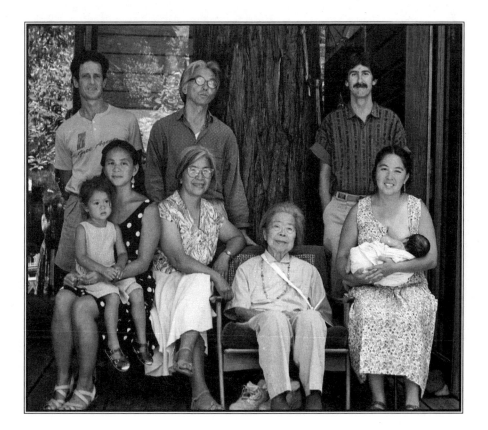

You, in me. Now you *and* me.

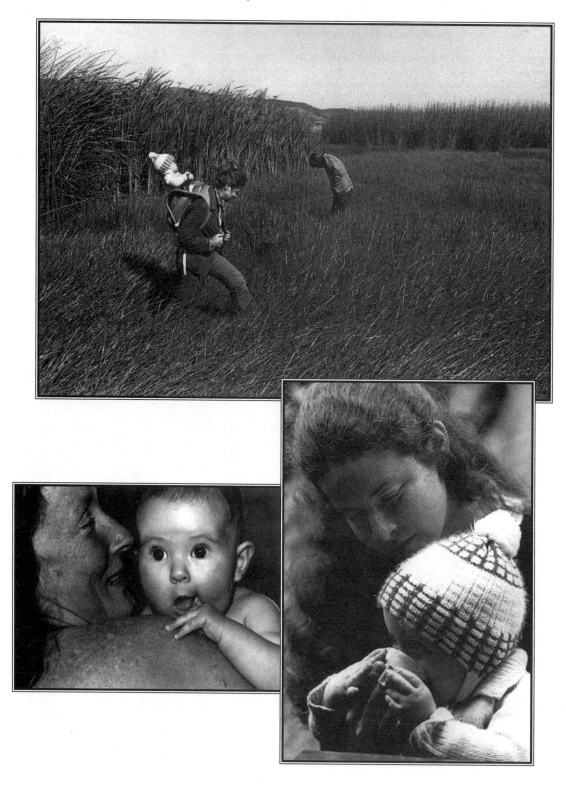

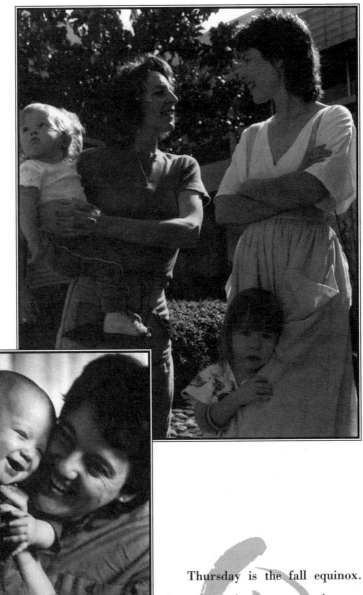

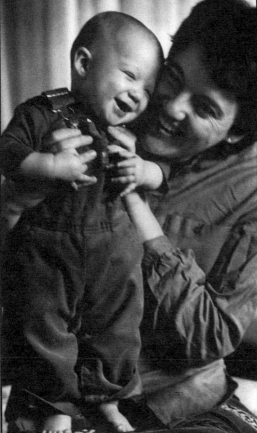

Thursday is the fall equinox. Susan invited us to a women's ceremony tonight to celebrate the earth and the changing of seasons. It's a whole new world for you.

RECOMMENDED RESOURCES

Pregnancy & Preparation for Birth:

A Celebration of Birth, by Sheila Kitzinger, Seattle, WA: Pennypress, Inc., 1986, or any other title by this author.

Active Birth: The New Approach To Giving Birth Naturally, by Janet Balaskas, Boston: Harvard Commons Press, 1992. Also look at other titles by this author.

Gentle Birth Choices, produced by Barbara Harper, RN. A 60-minute video showing natural births in a variety of settings, with different kinds of practitioners, including water birth, available through Global Maternal/Child Health Association, P.O. Box 366, West Linn, OR 97068, Tel: (800) 641-2229 or (503) 682-3600. See also her book by the same title, Rochester, VT: Inner Traditions, 1994.

Homebirth: The Essential Guide to Giving Birth Outside of the Hospital, by Sheila Kitzinger, New York: Dorling Kindersley, Inc., 1991.

Women Giving Birth: The Dutch Way of Birth, by Limburg and Smulders, Berkeley, CA: Celestial Arts, 1992.

Labor & Postpartum Care for Mothers:

After the Baby's Birth: A Woman's Way To Wellness, by Robin Lim, Berkeley, CA: Celestial Arts, 1991.

Mamatoto: A Celebration of Birth, by Carroll Dunham and The Body Shop, New York: Penguin Books, 1991.

Mothering the Mother: How a Doula Can Help You Have a Shorter, Easier, and Healthier Birth, by Klaus, Klaus, and Kennell, Reading, MA: Addison-Wesley, 1993.

Especially for Fathers:

Pregnant Fathers, by Jack Heinowitz, San Diego, CA: Parents As Partners Press, 1994, 4019 Goldfinch St., Suite 170, San Diego, CA 92103, Tel: (619) 234-7272, $12.95 + $2.00 shipping.

Being A Father: Family, Work, and Self, by *Mothering Magazine*, Santa Fe, NM: John Muir Publications, 1990.

Baby & Child Care and Development:

Bestfeeding: Getting Breastfeeding Right for You, by Renfrew, Arms, and Fisher, Berkeley, CA: Celestial Arts, 1990.

Circumcision, by *Mothering* magazine, Santa Fe, NM: John Muir Publications, 1988.

The Continuum Concept: Allowing Human Nature to Work Successfully, by Jean Liedloff, Reading, MA: Addison-Wesley, 1977.

Family Bed: An Age-Old Concept in Child Rearing, by Tine Thevenin, Garden City Park, NY: Avery Publishing Group, 1987. See also her book *Mothering and Fathering*.

Growing Together: A Parent's Guide To Baby's First Year, William Sears, M.D., Schaumburg, IL: La Leche League International, 1987. Look for his other books, too.

Infant Massage, by Vimala Schneider McClure, New York: Bantam, 1989. Also look for *The Tao of Motherhood* by the same author.

The Intelligence of Babies. An hour-long video with David Chamberlain and Suzanne Arms, focusing on consciousness of babies and life in the womb, distributed by Touch the Future, 4350 Lime Ave., Long Beach, CA 90807, Tel: (310) 426-2627, $24.00 + $3.00 shipping.

Touchpoints: Your Child's Emotional and Behavioral Development, by T. Berry Brazelton, Reading, MA: Addison-Wesley, 1992.

You Are Your Child's First Teacher, by Rahima Baldwin, Berkeley, CA: Celestial Arts, 1989.

Magazines:

Mothering, P.O. Box 1690, Santa Fe, NM 87504, Tel: (800) 827-1061. Providing information on alternatives in birth and parenting, midwifery, vaginal birth after cesarean, family health care, as well as natural remedies, baby-friendly toys, cotton diapers and baby and children's clothing, breastfeeding, lambskins, soft baby carriers, and earth-friendly products.

To find an independent birth educator or labor coach (doula):

ASPO Lamaze, 1840 Wilson Blvd., Suite 204, Arlington, VA 22201, Tel: (703) 524-7802.

Birthworks, 42 Tallwood Drive, Medford, NJ 08255, Tel: (609) 953-9380.

Bradley Childbirth (American Academy of Husband-Coached Childbirth), P.O. Box 5224, Sherman Oaks, CA 91413, Tel: (800) 423-2397.

Informed Birth and Parenting, P.O. Box 3675, Ann Arbor, MI 48106, Tel: (313) 662-6857.

International Childbirth Education Association (ICEA), P.O. Box 20048, Minneapolis, MN 55420, Tel: (612) 854-8660.

National Association of Childbirth Assistants, 265 Meridian Avenue, Suite 7, San Jose, CA 95123, Tel: (800) 868-6222.

To find a midwife, physician, or psychotherapist supporting natural childbirth and concerned with the sensitivity and consciousness of babies, or to learn about conferences and workshops:

The American College of Nurse-Midwives (ACNM), 818 Connecticut Ave. NW, Suite 900, Washington, DC 20006, Tel: (202) 728-9860.

International Cesarean Awareness Network (ICAN, formerly the Cesarean Prevention Movement), P.O. Box 276, Charles Summit, PA 18411, Tel: (717) 585-4226.

Midwives Alliance of North America (MANA), P.O. Box 175, Newton, KS, 67114, Tel: (316) 283-4543.

National Holistic Health Directory (thousands of physicians and other health practitioners listed in the U.S.), Dept. M, 342 Western Avenue, Brighton, MA 02135, $5.95.

The Association for Pre- and Perinatal Psychology & Health of North America, 1600 Prince Street, Suite 500, Alexandria, VA 22314, Tel: (703) 548-2802.

To find a birth center near you or help start one:

National Association of Childbearing Centers, RD 1, Box 1, Perkiomenville, PA 18074, Tel: (215) 234-1140.

To order almost any books or videos on the subjects in this book:

Cascade Healthcare & Birth & Life Bookstore, P.O. Box 12203, Salem, OR 97309, Tel: (800) 443-9942.

La Leche League International Catalog, for books, tapes, videos, posters, pamphlets, and breast pumps, Tel: (708) 519-7730.

Other Books and Films by Suzanne Arms:

Adoption: A Handful of Hope, Berkeley, CA: Celestial Arts, 1988. A compassionate exploration of the long-term impact of adoption upon adoptees, birth parents, and adoptive parents told through a series of true stories. Its emphasis is on openness and honesty in adoption, and the need for birth family and adoptive family to remain in contact, for the benefit of everyone involved.

Five Women, Five Births, a classic 28-minute video in black-and-white about choices and decisions, distributed by Informed Birth and Parenting, P.O. Box 3675, Ann Arbor, MI 48106, Tel: (313) 662-6857.
A moving portrait of five women, done using still photos with voice-over candid, intimate interviews suitable for any audience, including students and young children.

Immaculate Deception: A Fresh Look At Childbirth (with over 200 photos in black-and-white and color by the author), Berkeley, CA: Celestial Arts, 1994.
This is a totally new edition of the book named "A Best Buy of the Year" and called "Essential reading for any woman having a baby in an American hospital" by *The New York Times*. Weaving together history, anthropology, true stories, and narrative, it offers both a rationale and a blueprint for humane change [in how women and babies are cared for before, during, and after birth].

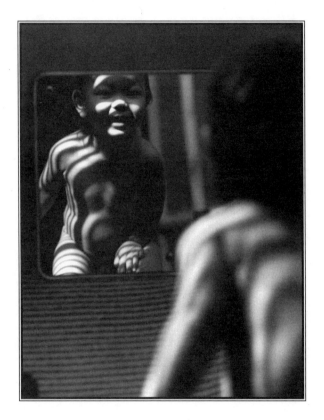